AGING
BRILLIANTLY

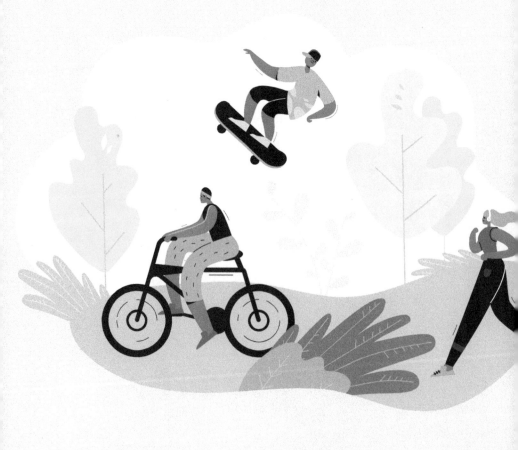

AGING
BRILLIANTLY

How to Eat, Move, Rest,
and Socialize Your Way
to Long Life

Dr. Patricia Pimentel Selassie

**ROCKRIDGE
PRESS**

Interior & Cover Designer: Peatra Jariya
Art Producer: Tom Hood
Editor: Rochelle Torke
Production Editor: Rachel Taenzler
Illustrations: iStock/Tera Vector, cover & pp. vi, 2; iStock/AnnaSivak, p. ii; iStock/ilyaliren, pp. viii, 8; iStock/grivina, pp. xii, 8, 22, 117; iStock/Ponomariova_Maria, pp. 11, 102; iStock/ UnitoneVector, pp. 12, 26, 69; iStock/Rassco, p. 14; iStock/Egor Shabanov, p. 16; iStock/ Invincible_bulldog, p. 36; iStock/Color_Life, p. 47; iStock/leila_divine, p. 52; istock/Svetlana Malysheva, p. 84; iStock/Volodymyr Kryshtal, p. 95; iStock/Anastasiia_New, p. 109;

Author Photo © Andreea Burciu-Ballen

ISBN: Print 978-1-64611-370-5 | eBook 978-1-64611-371-2
R0

To my beautiful mother,
Myrna Mata Pimentel,
who exudes grace,
intelligence, purpose, caring,
and adventure as she enjoys
her long and blessed life.

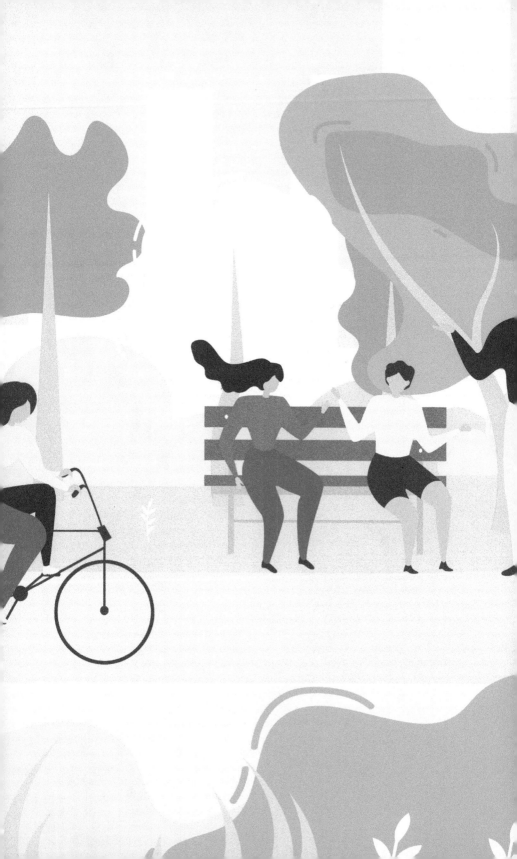

CONTENTS

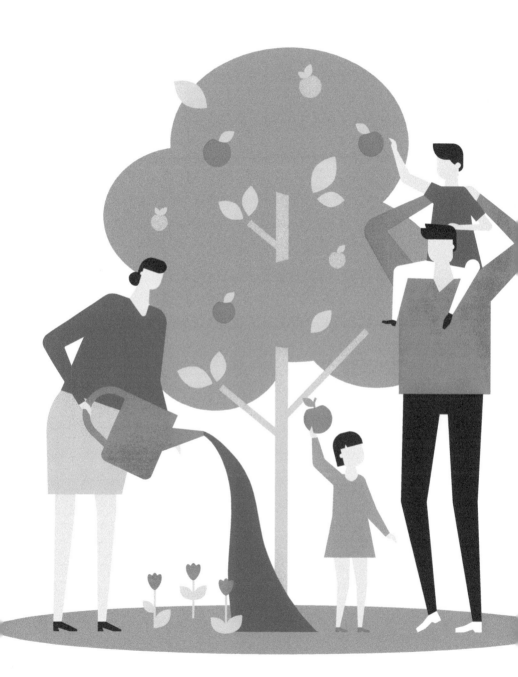

INTRODUCTION

My grandmother, Florecita Santiago Pimentel, was blessed to live 102 amazing years. My *lola*, which means "grandmother" in Tagalog, was a pharmacist in the Philippines. She gave birth to my father under an umbrella in the jungle during the Second World War. When their beloved hometown was invaded by the Japanese, she and my grandfather, a medical doctor, fled to the mountains with a donkey cart full of medicine, saving their own lives and, ultimately, the lives of many others. Lola's husband and her firstborn son, my dad, died before her, which devastated her but never broke her spirit.

She was full of positivity and laughter—a lot of laughter—the kind that made tears come to your eyes. She could be loud but was always loving and affectionate. Lola loved everyone she met, and they loved her back. Once, when talking about my maternal grandmother, she smiled and said, "Oh! She is my compadre, my friend." When talking about my dad's best friend, she would say, "I just looooong to see him." She really meant every word.

Definitely a proud woman, Lola lovingly chided my Jamaican husband by saying that she knows the mangos in Jamaica are delicious, but the Philippines has the very best. Every talent of her 19 grandchildren and countless great-grandchildren was always attributed to her side of the family. She loved to pray for us. And I often think that any blessing in my life is because of her.

Lola was generous with her time, very social, and extremely loyal. The last time I saw her, she was 92 years old, wearing black Versace jeans, and texting on her smartphone. My grandmother kept up with the times. That day she met our first daughter, then four years old. In her unique and spiritual way, she wrote out a prayer for our family on a piece of legal-size paper and read it aloud. Her prayer was so powerful that day,

I felt as though she put a force field of protection around our family.

My name is Dr. Patricia Pimentel Selassie, and I'm a naturopathic doctor, wife, mother of five beautiful daughters, and resident of New York City. I was blessed to have so much time with my lola and am so grateful today watching my mother relish being a grandmother after twice surviving cancer.

My goal is to follow their legacy and live a long rich life. However, my grandfather and father died early—both in their forties—due to heart disease and cancer, respectively. Genetically, I seem to have inherited a roulette wheel of longevity and health possibilities. So, what does my destiny hold?

And, more importantly, which fate will I create for myself through my own effort, beliefs, and choices?

I've witnessed my patients heal and come back from diabetes, heart disease, obesity, thyroid disorder, skin problems, autoimmune disease, Crohn's disease, ulcerative colitis, GERD, fibroids—you name it—and go on to live incredibly full lives. In some cases, it takes great determination. At other times, they accomplished great healing through relatively small and simple lifestyle changes.

When I came across journalist Dan Buettner's coverage of the Blue Zones, parts of the world famous for longevity and robust aging, the research he illuminated mirrored my own observations as a healer. Centenarians in the Blue Zones practice some of the same habits that naturopathic medicine encourages: a diet of unprocessed foods and a focus on relationships, community, faith, and purpose.

Naturopathic medicine also encourages *vis medicatrix naturae*, which is Latin for the "healing power of nature" and/or the "innate, natural ability of the body to heal itself." Healing from illness and aging powerfully are two processes that employ similar methods and choices. Those personal habits are what we'll explore in this book.

WHY THIS BOOK?

I was inspired to write this book because there's mounting evidence that particular lifestyle choices, no matter where you come from, seem to lead to "more life." I define this as a longer, stronger, and more continuously robust life. I hope this book informs, inspires, and empowers you to try on these helpful habits—and celebrate and share the healthy choices you've already made. May it become your "super ager's guide to the galaxy," a tool for you to return to again and again as you become the master of your own vitality and designer of your own graceful aging path.

The first part of the book will arm you with powerful information on aging well. The second half will help you translate those insights into actions. *Aging Brilliantly* aims to help you put more life in your years, your body, and your brain.

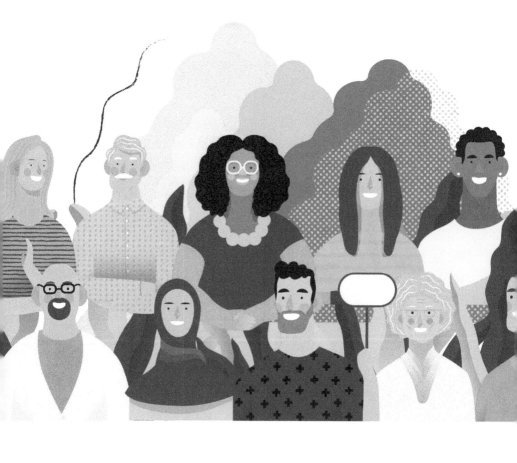

WHO AGES WELL AND WHY

For my centenarian grandmother, faith was a priority—and if longevity research is right, it may have contributed to her long life. For others, longevity boosters might be a diet filled with vegetables and an exercise routine they find challenging and enjoyable. When looking for the keys to long-term vitality and extended life, much of our research is turning toward communities known worldwide for their masterful aging and long lives. In this chapter, we'll explore some of those regions and what they have to teach us about why some humans thrive well into their golden years.

As you'll see, no matter where you live, aging well has some universal components we can all adopt. Let's explore those lessons—and prepare for action.

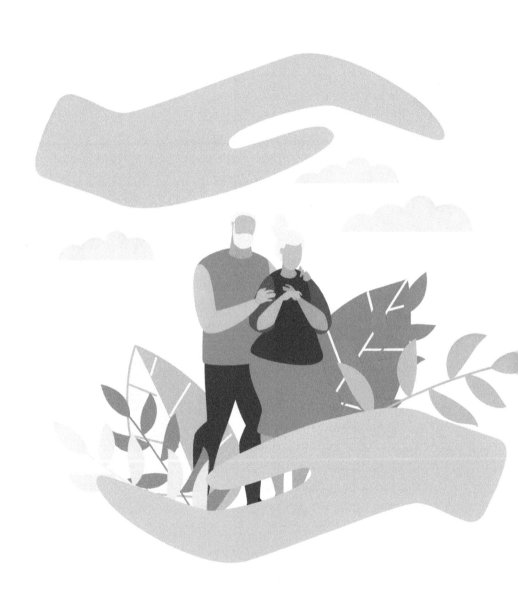

CHAPTER 1

Lessons
from the People
Who Live Longest

When creating our own strategies for aging gracefully and powerfully, it's great to start by studying the masters, the people who live long and well. I'm speaking about the residents of the "Blue Zones." The Blue Zones gained notoriety when *National Geographic* journalist Dan Buettner began covering them in 2005. In these regions, not only do we find high numbers of centenarians—people who live to age 100 or beyond—we also find older people living with great energy and stamina, who complete challenging physical tasks alongside much younger people.

LIVING LONG AND WELL

There are five Blue Zones in the world: Okinawa, Japan; Sardinia, Italy; Ikaria, Greece; the Nicoya Peninsula, Costa Rica; and Loma Linda, California. Yes, there is a Blue Zone here in the United States. I find it reassuring that, in a country known for obesity and chronic illnesses, it's still quite possible to live a long, robust life.

There are some common lifestyle habits we can observe in these master agers:

- A diet abundant in vegetables: carrots, tomatoes, onions, greens, and eggplant, as well as plant-based proteins like fava or black beans

- Exercise or physical work, including lifting heavy things, as a part of everyday life

- An emphasis on family, friends, and relatives

- A tendency to serve a community of which they feel a part

- A sense of humor and buoyant enjoyment of life

We'll explore these communities and other longevity research throughout the book, but here's a snapshot of life in a few Blue Zones to get us started:

Okinawa

Longevity is admired and elders are valued as spiritual leaders in Okinawa, Japan. This status gives them a strong sense of purpose. There is also an emphasis on maintaining lifelong friendships. Okinawans practice healthy habits like eating light, gardening, and praying.

Sardinia

The Sardinian greeting *a kent'annos* means "health and life for 100 years." Predominantly sheepherders by trade, Sardinian centenarians value physical work and family. Workdays start early and include tending to animals and walking up to four miles before the midday meal. At lunchtime, they have a glass of local red wine rich in polyphenols, which, according to a review of studies published in *Molecules*, may play a role in preventing cardiovascular disease. They pair the wine with pecorino cheese, a cheese rich in omega-3 fatty acids, fats known to prevent inflammation in the body.

Loma Linda

Many residents of this California town are members of the Seventh-day Adventist Church. Followers of this religion are often quite committed to their faith, which includes eating a vegetarian diet. The combination is a winning formula for the people of Loma Linda, who are ten times more likely to live to 100 than other Americans. As members of the same church, they attend many social events and report experiencing a strong sense of community. Social connection and purpose are common characteristics of this population.

Nicoya

The Nicoya Peninsula of Costa Rica is a topographically beautiful place filled with wild flora and fauna. Wild monkeys swing above the hiking trails that sometimes double as roads. Fresh mangos and other nutritious fruit hang from the trees. The *tico* (as native Costa Ricans are called) diet consists of fresh food that grows or grazes on the local farms and ranches. Like families in the other Blue Zones, tico families work hard and work together, with a shared sense of purpose, to serve their community. In Dan Buettner's book *The Blue Zones*, one researcher, Dr. Xinia Fernandez-Rojas, observed:

"We notice that the most highly functioning people over 90 in Nicoya have a few common traits. One of them is that they feel a strong sense of service to others or care for their family. We see that as soon as they lose this, the switch goes off. They die very quickly if they don't feel needed."

WHAT DOES DNA HAVE TO DO WITH IT?

Our DNA is often compared to a blueprint. The DNA in our genes make proteins that perform certain functions in the body to, hopefully, keep you healthy.

Whether your genes support you or work against you is highly determined by your lifestyle. Doctors once believed that your DNA was your destiny, an inexorable map of how your physical life would play out. It turns out that—short of a few genetic mutations that directly cause disease—much of the rest of our DNA can be influenced by our behavior. Epigenetics is the study of gene expression, and how our own choices can ignite or turn off a particular outcome. One study from 2015 looking at centenarians suggests that longevity is one-third attributed to genes and two-thirds attributed to epigenetics and environment. Another study, on identical twins, finds that longevity is 20 percent dictated by our genes and 80 percent dictated by our lifestyle.

For example, we know some superfoods with high antioxidant levels appear to turn on cancer-fighting genes and turn off the inflammation that contributes to aging. A study completed at the National University of Natural Medicine in Portland, Oregon, concluded that "specific superfoods, such as blueberries, have a protective epigenetic effect." In fact, people living in the Blue Zones are simply living in a culture that promotes successful lifestyle habits that include eating certain superfoods. These time-tested habits, passed down effortlessly by their ancestors, are turning on their longevity genes, rather than leaving their DNA to act as the final arbiter of health.

MOVE: USE YOUR BODY EVERY DAY

Marge Jetton was a centenarian living in Loma Linda, California. After rising early and saying her prayers each day, Marge
walked one mile, lifted weights in the exercise room of her
senior living quarters, and rode for six to eight miles on the stationary bike. She did this each day of her life with the exception
of the Sabbath, a day of rest as practiced by her religion. She
also tended the community garden where she resided.

"If it's healthy, I'm all for it," Marge said. She stayed active
and positive with her mantra of "use it or lose it!" Even in her
90s, Marge drove her car, volunteered at the senior center,
and kept a hair appointment every Friday. Marge's life was a
recipe for aging gracefully. She passed away in 2011 at the
age of 106.

On the other side of the world, Sardinian shepherds often
walk their sheep through four to six miles of rocky terrain. Their
morning walk is equivalent to walking three and a half miles
in two hours, bowling or golfing, or gardening for hours. They
eat from fruit and olive trees and get together for family and
community dinners.

The American lifestyle can be very sedentary. However, if we
want to live long, robust lives, it's important to find ways to use
our bodies and challenge ourselves every day. Many Americans
may not have sheep to herd, so we need to make it a point to
move our bodies daily.

Since our daily activity may not naturally contain much
movement, injecting new ways to use our bodies in our everyday
life is a must. Rather than accepting that technology makes us
sedentary and neglectful of our bodies, it can be fun to challenge ourselves to defy this notion. Doing some physical activity
for less than an hour each day can pay huge dividends in our
energy levels and the way we look.

In chapter 2, we will discuss different ways we can incorporate movement into your lives. Most centenarian studies
find that thriving older people regularly practice low-intensity

exercises as they go about their daily activities. A report published in the *British Journal of Sports Medicine* followed 1,180 men with an average age of 78 for five years. The study found that it was the overall volume of exercise that mattered most to longevity, meaning that the more time they spent being active in some way each week, the healthier they were. In addition, "low intensity" is a winning idea because part of living long is preserving joints that would otherwise wear out if constantly overexerted.

EAT REAL FOOD: GREAT-GREAT-GRANDMA STYLE

A common thread among those living longer is a diet rich in whole and unprocessed foods. Many naturopathic doctors prescribe a diet like the ones our great-great-grandmothers would have eaten. Processed foods are a relatively new phenomenon. Much of our modern diets are filled with foods created for convenience, and nutrition seems to be an afterthought. People are running on snacks in bags, protein or granola bars, and premade, sugary smoothies served in bottles. These foods spike blood sugar and offer limited nutritional value.

Listed below are some of the meals traditionally consumed in high-longevity communities:

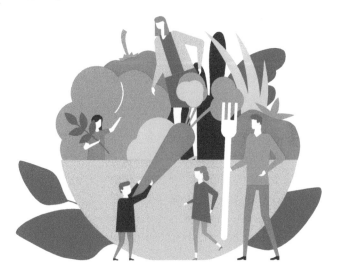

Okinawa, Japan: fermented unprocessed soybeans, cabbage, fish, homegrown vegetables

Nicoya, Costa Rica: black beans, maize, eggs, tropical fruit

Sardinia, Italy: fava beans, vegetables, small amounts of fish or eggs, pecorino cheese

Loma Linda, California: a mostly vegetarian diet with plenty of beans and vegetables

Crete, Greece: olive oil (up to six teaspoons per day), vegetables, vegetable dips like fava bean pâté or eggplant and garlic dip

The Kuna from Panama: Cocoa, plantains, yucca, corn, kidney beans, and locally grown fruit

CONNECT: RELATIONSHIPS, FAMILY, AND SPIRITUAL SUPPORT

A connection with others is imperative for longevity. Those who age well often place a strong focus on relationships, family ties, community relations, and spiritual faith. Connection goes hand in hand with a sense of purpose. Contributing to one's family or community gives people a reason to wake up in the morning. Thankfully, even if you are shy and find yourself lonely and without family, there are countless ways you can plug in. Centenarian Marge Jetton agreed.

"It took me a year [after her husband died] to realize that the world wasn't going to come to me. That's when I started volunteering again, and it was the best thing to ever happen to me. I found that when you are depressed, that's when you do something for somebody else."

Humans don't often reach 100 years of age while living in isolation. They not only have people around them, the people surrounding them value their contribution.

RELAX: WE AREN'T BUILT FOR CONSTANT STRESS

A special consideration for most people living in the industrialized world is how to lower stress levels. In American society, there seems to be a pervasive attitude that working more and making more money is how we achieve "success." However, if a long, healthy, peaceful life is your objective, you have to curtail stress. Stress can be linked to almost every single chronic disease. Studies show that chronic stress in particular compromises the immune system and causes damage to multiple organs and tissues. In order to put more life in your years, we need reminders for self-care, relaxation, and even the simple act of breathing.

Cultures that observe a Sabbath day, a day just for rest, put a focused effort into slowing down once a week. The Orthodox Jewish community and the Seventh-day Adventist Christians both take an entire day of rest each week. They have one more day of rest and recovery than their American counterparts. As fifty-two Sabbath days occur in a year, that is almost the equivalent of two months' rest. In *The Blue Zones*, Randy Roberts, a Seventh-day Adventist pastor, echoes the need for downtime:

"I've heard over and over again from students in rigorous programs like medicine and dentistry, and from faculty, too, that they can't wait for the Sabbath to come because they have a guilt-free time when they don't have to study or do some other obligation. They can just be with their family and friends and with God, and just relax and rejuvenate."

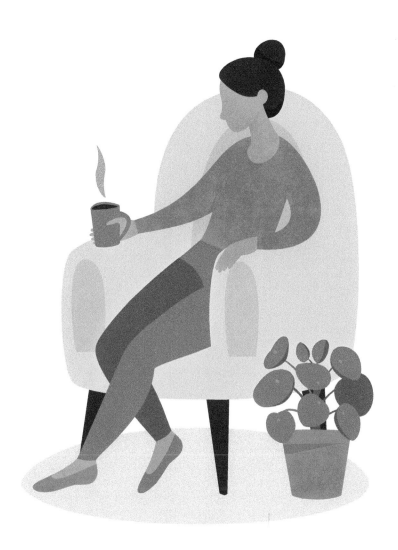

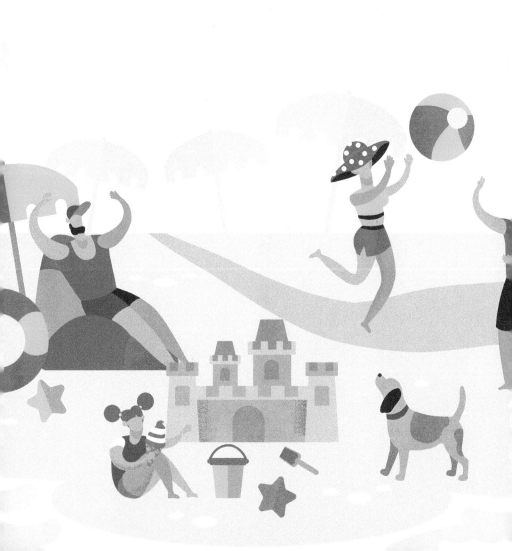

LET'S DO THIS

T here are habits human beings can adopt which will help us achieve longevity and years of vitality. The next four chapters represent the four pillars to become a master ager. These four pillars are move, eat real food, connect, and relax. After each chapter, you will have the opportunity to take an in-depth look at the current lifestyles of master agers, and see how you can take action to begin new habits for longevity with vitality.

To become a master ager, one must practice every day. Eventually you will become so proficient in living a life that leads to vitality and longevity that it actually becomes a part of your identity. Masterful aging requires dedication, repetition, and practice. However, everyone has the power to make these changes. At the end of each of the next four chapters are the Recap and Quick Tips sections and a Self-Assessment section. Pick one or two of the takeaways or insights from each chapter and put them into action.

After completing the self-assessment at the end of each section, readers will establish a baseline for their current health. Consider repeating the self-assessment 30 to 90 days later to check your progress. Please review the Recap and Quick Tips to add even more beneficial lifestyle changes into your daily life. Mastering these pillars may lead to many years of feeling vital, purposeful, joyful, and even proud. The goal is to enjoy more than 100 years of life.

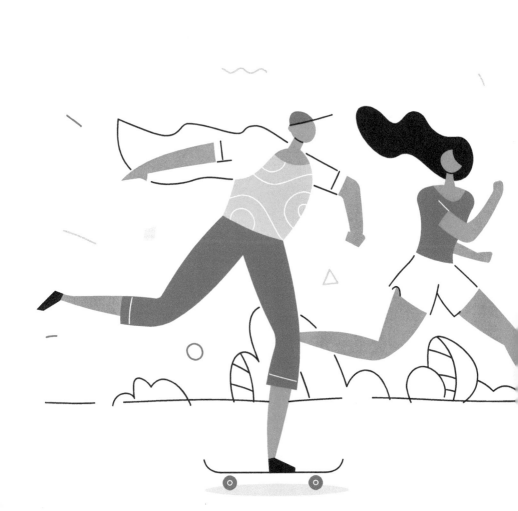

CHAPTER 2

Move

S trength and mobility directly contribute to vitality and over-all quality of life. In this chapter, I'll explain why it's so important to avoid the frail trail by protecting every aspect of your body by staying fit and active.

The most common excuse for lack of exercise is lack of time. In actuality, the inverse is true: We don't have time to neglect exercise, because exercise adds years to our lives. Today, it is important and urgent enough for us to steal time to exercise. The more we make exercise a priority and incorporate it into our daily lives, the higher dividends it will pay in joint, bone, endo-crine, and mental health. The older we get, the more important it is to make sure exercise has solidified its place in our daily routine.

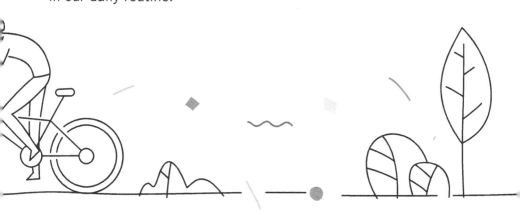

OUR BODIES ARE DESIGNED TO MOVE

The human body is designed to move often and in different ways, like climbing, bending, lifting, pushing, pulling, throwing, jumping, and carrying heavy objects from here to there.

For millions of years, humans depended on their strong bodies every day. From sunrise until bedtime, movement in a hunter/gatherer society was innate and necessary. Working with others often required long trips to trade goods, for example. Our ancestors may have walked many miles over many days in order to meet with neighboring tribes.

As agriculture took hold and humans lived in more permanent settlements and villages, they remained active, migrating with the seasons, plowing fields, planting, caring for animals, harvesting, and hoisting themselves onto horses. Soldiers wore cumbersome body armor and carried heavy weapons. Women carried babies on their backs all day while gathering food or tending crops. They did laundry by beating clothing against river rocks. Without the ease of hopping in the car, they instead

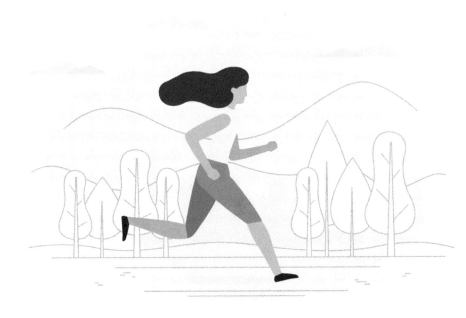

walked long distances. Without supermarkets or daily deliveries, our ancestors raised crops and dug wells for water. We were constantly squatting, standing, reaching, running, and walking. After millions of years of activity, the past 500 years—and the past 100 in particular—delivered a remarkable new invention: sedentary life. That experiment isn't going too well, but we'll come back to that shortly.

THE LONGEST-LIVING PEOPLE TODAY ARE ACTIVE

Today's centenarians of the world tend to live more like our ancestors. Their physically active lives are a force of habit, local culture, and necessity. For example, before noon each day, farmers in Sardinia have completed most of their physical chores and have walked a few miles. Okinawans have already risen from their floor dozens of times where they sit, without furniture, on mats. Even very old Okinawans have walked to a friend's house or worked in their garden.

In modern American life, many of us have occupations that require long hours in a chair. In these cases, our bodies are healthiest when we try to mimic the movements of ancient people. Standing up from our desks every 20 minutes is imperative to keep the blood flow running to our brain, joints, and extremities.

Ideally, 10-minute breaks may be spent taking vigorous walks. Office workers can take walking meetings now when they need to meet in a small group. Others take calls as they walk around their office building. A CEO who frequents my medical practice says he does bicep curls when he is on the phone. If there's a physical chore that needs to be done at the office, volunteer for it. Loading the water cooler or putting away dishes is a great break from the sitting. Of course, use caution when lifting heavy objects—especially if you haven't been lifting much lately—but with each bit of physical work you add to your day, you're conditioning your body for a lifetime of energy, strength, muscle, joint, and bone health.

YOUR MUSCLES, JOINTS, AND BONES ARE YOUR BEST FRIENDS

Few people know that muscles are as vital as organs. Muscle atrophy—the shrinking and weakening of our muscles—can create serious health challenges. As we age, we naturally begin to lose muscle mass. When muscles diminish significantly, we call the condition sarcopenia. Sarcopenia is a serious situation that leads to a loss in balance, an unsteady gait, and, possibly, decreased life expectancy. Older adults may notice that simple acts like opening jars, carrying groceries, standing up from a chair, or lifting grandchildren have become more difficult. Their arms may fatigue swiftly. This loss of power is called dynapenia, and it affects the ability to perform activities of daily living. If these small tasks challenge you, that's your cue to spring into action and begin to repair your muscles and regain your youthful vitality.

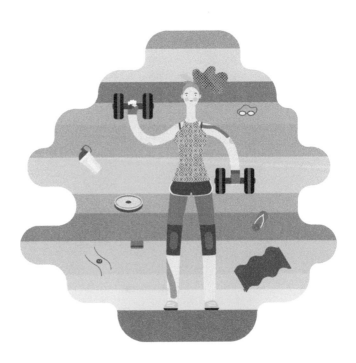

Strong muscles are also your insurance against mobility chal-lenges. They decrease wear and tear on your spine, bones, and joints; encourage more youthful hormone levels; and protect your metabolism from slowing down. There's also a connec-tion between muscle strength—particularly in the legs—and brain mass and reduced dementia risk. We'll cover that in more detail soon.

For now, understand that frequent movement and the habit of challenging your muscles is critical to various bodily func-tions. In this way, through muscle mass and strength, you can protect your balance, mobility, metabolism, hormones, and brain.

Hip fractures are common in senior populations and are most often caused by a loss of agility and balance. For older adults, hip fractures can be quite serious, resulting in long recovery times or, unfortunately, complications like infections or blood clots. About 95 percent of hip fractures are due to falls alone. The positive news is that they can be completely prevented. We can indeed protect our bodies by adding strength training to our daily routine. Balance-building exercises like yoga and Pilates and simple stretching can also be vital in the prevention of falls by increasing flexibility. These exercises keep the body elas-tic and in balance, both physically and mentally. Consistently building muscle through movement ensures our bodies retain our muscle, bone, and joint health.

Speaking of joints, it's important to note that, like the rest of our bodies, our joints were designed to move. As we age, there is wear and tear on the joint, sometimes leading to aches and pains. People sometimes make the mistake of thinking it is best to keep still. However, there is not a strong blood supply going into the joint. You will need to move the joint to pump nutrition into it. So if we were used to exercising before pain in our joints occurred, using our joints during recovery would be much easier. Like the rest of your body, your joints are meant to be used. Lack of exercise speeds up their deterioration just like other body parts. Let's take a look at how your body benefits from movement.

AGE STRONG:
THE MANY WAYS TO KEEP UP YOUR STRENGTH

As I've mentioned, modern life can be quite sedentary. In a typical day, people often go from bed to the breakfast table, then from the car to their office desks, and back home to sit at the dinner table. Sometimes before dinner, there's a stop to sit at the bar for happy hour. However, after dinner many of us migrate to the couch before we lie down again for the night.

Thus, it's important to decide how you'll seek out movement and keep up your strength. The good news is that, when you really look, the opportunities are endless and the flavors of exercise and movement are vast.

Exercising with others or joining a community fitness program can have the added bonus of creating a new social outlet. The people you meet, and the class schedule itself, should keep you engaged and enthused. Attending a regular fitness class can become a ritual you look forward to, not a chore. If you don't look forward to your class, you haven't found the right one yet. You'll need to find a class that isn't too advanced for your current fitness level and features attainable movement options as well as music and an atmosphere you enjoy. Check your local listings. Many community centers, libraries, and hospitals offer low-cost or free fitness classes.

If a gym or group class is out of reach, remember that strength and resistance training can be accomplished at home by simply doing push-ups or lifting small weights (like cans or cartons of milk) before bed or during your morning routine. There are many fitness instructors and classes on the Internet; you can always follow along in front of your laptop.

Ideally, your exercise routine will include strategies to improve balance, flexibility, and cardiovascular exercise to strengthen the heart muscle. Just remember that the best type of exercise is the exercise that you actually do—and look forward to. It stands to reason that if you do something you enjoy, you're more likely to do it regularly.

Stick with what works for you, just make it a goal to keep leveling up. But it's always fun to try something new, as well. You can create a workout that functions for you in the moment—for example: Go to your daughter's hip-hop class, try a barre toning class, learn an ancient art like tai chi, or play a game like pickleball. These different types of movement will not only work out different muscle groups, they'll become rituals you look forward to as you start to experience the mood and energy boost they deliver.

A quick important note: Exercise is always good. However, if you have chronic fatigue or are dealing with a serious health challenge, you may need to leave interval training, weight lifting, and vigorous exercise alone. Gentle, stress-free exercise like walking in nature, tai chi, or restorative yoga will be more appropriate for you.

Walking

Our bodies are designed for walking. Many doctors and trainers consider walking to be the most complete full-body exercise. Almost everyone can do it. It's free and no special equipment is needed. A brisk walk is low impact, and normally, does not overstress the joints. It can be done in the country, the city, or anywhere in between, at most any time of year. We can do it in the gym, a park, a mall, or simply by heading out the front door. We control the pace and the place. Walking keeps legs toned and requires no special training. Be vigilant about posture by making sure you point your feet straight ahead for a steady gait. Walking is also a great way to simply get you where you're going, such as when you're running errands. It's beneficial whether it's a 15-minute walk to the subway or a couple of miles as a break in the day.

Hiking

I went to medical school in Seattle, Washington, which is full of amazing hiking trails. My med school friends would come down off the mountains, looking refreshed even while carrying loads of backpacks, trail maps, reusable water bottles, and stainless-steel coffee cups. This was a new idea for me. It was intimidating as I thought they must be hard-core health and fitness nuts. Then one day, while studying in a café, a friend suggested a short hike as a study break.

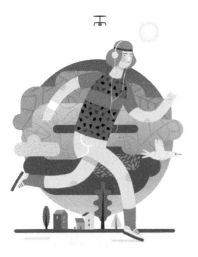

"I'm wearing a dress. I don't have any trail mix on me!" I protested immediately.

"Don't be silly, a hike is just a code word for taking a walk in nature," she replied.

Needless to say, we went on that 10-minute hike, and I have been a hiker ever since. As always, check with your doctor if you have any physical injuries or special circumstances, but for the most part, anyone can become a hiker. It's just a matter of knowing your fitness level and picking the right trail for you. Being in nature has its own set of spiritual and mental benefits, but the physical benefits of hiking cannot be overstated. Hiking improves bone, brain, muscle, and adrenal health, as you will read in the coming chapters.

High Intensity Interval Resistance Training (HIIRT)

It sounds intense. How can anything pronounced "hurt" be good for you? In reality, this type of exercise is less intimidating and more accessible than you might think. It's a fancy way of saying "move your body a lot of different ways and get your heart rate up from time to time while you're at it." HIIRT training can increase strength, balance, muscle, and cardio quickly all in one session. These dynamic routines can flip on the switch to muscle building and thus, a fat-burning metabolism. How does it work?

For example, taking a HIIRT approach on a stationary bike means practicing short sprints to elevate the heart rate to a point at which the exercise is challenging and the breath labored. You can still make conversation but will feel a bit winded. Then, slow down but keep moving until you catch your breath and the heart rate slows a bit. Now, challenge the body to repeat the cycle again, but this time strap on some ankle weights to increase the challenge. This is the "resistance" part of the concept.

A version of this cycle of burst and rest can work for many of us—but remember to adapt it to your current fitness level. If you have not exercised for a long time, it's a good idea to consult with your doctor and possibly a trainer when starting this approach. Whether you're 25 or 75, this type of varied interval training, adjusted as needed, can deliver huge health benefits.

Going from a resting heart rate to a sprint and back again mimics the ancient human lifestyle—so it's what we're built for. Just remember that the definition of a sprint varies for each of us, but combining low- and high-intensity exercise can serve most bodies across a range of ages.

Weight Lifting

Many people conflate weight training with bodybuilding. Many of my female patients, for example, express concern about building muscle and "bulking up" at the suggestion of lifting heavy weights. In actuality, if done correctly, the opposite is true. Female bodybuilders look that way because they are most likely intentionally training and eating specifically to look that way. It is very difficult to accomplish that with simple weight training and healthy eating.

Load-bearing strength training is the most important type of exercise to build and strengthen muscles. It helps us not only prevent muscle atrophy, but to increase calorie-burning, bone-protecting muscle mass. As Dr. Deedra Mason, a colleague and fellow naturopathic doctor, tells her patients, "It is important to lift heavy things and put them back down." This is simply stated, yet very wise. Weight training will singularly contribute to longevity and a strong, lean, energetic body capable of a wide range of activities.

Tai Chi

This centuries-old Chinese body-mind exercise is an excellent form of movement, especially for seniors. Seniors, more than all other age groups, must be mindful of choosing safe exercise strategies. Tai chi is a very low-impact, slow form of martial arts. The movements help integrate mind, body, and breath, much like meditation. Tai chi creates a mindful energy, supports balance, helps manage stress, and increases flexibility.

A recent study looked at 90 sarcopenic men between the ages of 85 and 101 years of age. Some of the men were instructed in tai chi training for eight weeks while a control group received reminders not to increase their physical activity. After two months, the tai chi group scored higher on muscle strength, balance, and overall physical performance. How-tos on tai chi are readily available online, and many urban areas host morning tai chi groups in the park. As with any exercise, the more you can get outside for fresh air and time in nature, the better you'll feel.

Yoga

This movement option comes in a vast range of styles and intensity levels—from restorative to power yoga. It's generally low impact but can be challenging. Yoga is a series of poses that emphasize breath, balance, strength, and flexibility. By putting the body into a wide range of positions, you end up feeling rejuvenated, peaceful, and strong. Yoga strengthens the body by consistently challenging it to move in new directions.

Yoga classes may be a good place to start in building your community. If you are new to this type of exercise, start with a beginners' class. Be open with your instructor about any injuries or painful positions. If you are an advanced yogi, it often helps to try new classes to keep it fresh and enjoyable. Restorative yoga classes have the added benefit of helping alleviate the symptoms of stress, like insomnia or anxiety. For seniors, a chair yoga class may be the perfect starting point.

Pilates

Pilates was named after Joseph Pilates, who, in the 1920s, developed a set of exercises with ballerinas in mind. This specific set of movements emphasizes flexibility, muscular strength, toning, and endurance especially in the area of proper postural alignment and core strength.

Dance

There are so many types of dance to try: salsa, bachata, Zumba, ballroom, hip-hop, step, barre ballet, modern. The list is endless. In college, I took a ballroom dance class to fulfill a gym requirement. One evening, as part of an assignment, I found myself on the top floor of a hotel in a room filled with seniors. My ballroom class was mostly composed of young women, so the older gentlemen in the class had to work extra hard. One particular widower said to me:

"My wife was the most wonderful person in the world, but we never danced. She just wasn't into it. When she passed away, I was very depressed for a couple of years until one day, she came to me in a dream and told me to get off the couch and dance. I have been dancing every week and I love it. I am happy to dance and I am never short of a beautiful young woman to dance with. I will stay around in this life just to dance."

For regular exercisers, try changing up your routine with dancing to keep you from getting bored.

Swimming

Swimming is a gentle way to build strength and improve musculature with zero impact. Propelling oneself through the water burns calories and builds strength quickly using the natural resistance of water. It is excellent for people who have injuries from other sports, and the benefits of swimming and water movement are evident from the very first session. Swimming is less likely to cause injury, yet utilizes almost every muscle group, including the arms, legs, and core. These are engaged simultaneously and consistently. Water can also be emotionally therapeutic.

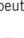

"Wake and Shake"

This set of exercises is particularly fun to do with children and seniors. Simply sit in a comfortable chair, hold your hands out in front of you, and shake them vigorously from the wrist. Do this for 20 to 30 seconds, then stop. Tune in and feel your blood vessels open and blood start circulating through your wrists, up into the hands, and down into your fingertips. Feel all the joints in your arms loosen up and readjust themselves. The burst of circulation and wellness that your hands experience is the same experience your whole body receives when you exercise.

Incidental Exercise

Adding little bits of movement and exertion throughout the day, without a gym, is a great way to protect your body. This is called incidental exercise and it can go a long way toward turning a sedentary life into a more active one. Consider your daily routine and ask where you could add some steps or other movement. For example, could you walk or bike to the store instead of drive? Carrying groceries, cleaning the house, and taking the stairs instead of the elevator are all chances to move. You can also set an alarm on your phone to stand up every hour. It all counts.

There was an important study published in *Diabetes Care* in October 2018 on the effects of interrupting a sedentary lifestyle with short (just three-minute) bouts of moderate physical activity. This study looked at 35 children who were overweight with sedentary lifestyles. They put the children into two different groups: a "sitting" group and a "sitting + walking" group. The children in the "sitting" group sat for 3 hours. The second group sat for the same amount of time, but every 30 minutes added 3 minutes of walking on a treadmill. Just that tiny amount of exercise—a total of 15 minutes done in 3-minute intervals—lowered their insulin secretion, thus improving their use of insulin and subsequently making it easier to lose weight. Theoretically, this small amount of movement can help prevent the development of diabetes.

Enjoy binge-watching Netflix? It doesn't have to be a sedentary pastime. Try getting up between episodes or during commercials and march in place for three minutes. Are you watching with kids? Have a dance party instead of screen time. Lunges and squats can be done anywhere at almost any time. One new mother I know spent most of her postpartum days lunging in place with the baby strapped securely to her chest in the baby carrier. From morning until evening she lunged through the kitchen, while online, and even while taking work calls. Her body bounced back from pregnancy and childbirth in record time, and she had more energy and stamina for her two older children. If you must remain sitting, try leg lifts from the couch or stretch out your arms and do a "wake and shake."

Vitality through Movement:
Stories from My Medical Practice

I have a patient I'll call Joshua who had a brain hemorrhage, a subsequent fall, and a terrible head injury. Digestive issues had plagued him for many years, even before the stroke. Today, Joshua gets up in the early hours of the day, stretches, and rides his stationary bike. He takes a walk outside before even the earliest NYC commuters come out. When I first started seeing him, he described his walks as sometimes frightening, as he felt weak and had what he called severe "energy drops." The work put in was arduous at first, but he stuck with it. He now couples his walks with a swim at a club close by. Then he hails a cab to take him back home. He sees these seemingly minor victories, like swimming and hailing a cab, as huge milestones. Each independent task helps him feel like he is fully living life again. Even more impressive, Joshua continues to oversee a successful business with many employees. He credits his dedication to exercise for his rapid recovery and continually improving health.

Another patient, David, used to weigh 400 pounds. He runs a garage for large trucks. When I first started working with him, he used lifestyle changes and sheer determination to lose 26 pounds. Soon we added regular exercise. He began by simply walking, then moved on to the stationary bike, and then started lifting with a personal trainer. The weight melted off. He now weighs under 300 pounds and is still losing inches.

A third patient of mine, Amelia, is a vibrant senior who incorporated a morning exercise ritual that has helped her improve almost every aspect of her daily life. She begins on her back for leg lifts and stretches. Then she marches in place and does arm exercises, squats, and push-ups. The entire ritual takes her less than 15 minutes. At the senior center, Amelia says she is more agile than almost all the other seniors. She is in the front of every exercise class and marvels at her mobility. Amelia is 87 years old.

THE MUSCLE-BRAIN CONNECTION

As I mentioned, research shows that there is a muscle-mind connection (MMC). This is the idea that when exercising, particularly when contracting a specific muscle like the biceps or a quad muscle, the muscles will improve their growth when the brain focuses on the action of lifting the weight, as opposed to thinking about anything else. When focusing on the weight and the muscle group, the brain activates the neuromuscular junction, where neurons are fired. After the neuromuscular junction is activated, it engages and recruits more muscle fibers. The muscle gets a better workout than it would have if you did not use your mind to focus on the exercise at hand.

In addition, some fascinating new research finds a correlation between muscle strength and cognitive performance in older adults. Leg strength in particular was associated with greater neural activity in the hippocampus, a brain area associated with dementia. So, in other words, older people with stronger legs also had a healthier, more active hippocampus, pointing again to the interconnectivity of the brain and muscles.

The take-home message is that we should definitely focus on exercise and growing our muscles as a tool in our brain health arsenal. So keep your legs and whole body fit and keep those neural pathways between your brain and body firing strong.

Other research shows that choosing a variety of exercises also helps improve brain function. Every time you take a different route on a daily walk, when you learn a new dance step or exercise routine, you improve brain health and stave off brain deterioration.

When discussing the brain-body connection, we also cannot neglect the power of endorphins. When we exercise, endorphins are released. Endorphins are chemicals produced by the brain to relieve stress and pain. Stress is associated with pretty much every chronic health issue. Simply put, the benefits of exercise are plentiful, and, if you want to live a healthy, long life, start moving and stay in motion.

TO RETIRE OR NOT RETIRE

Contrary to popular belief, a growing body of evidence suggests that putting off retirement might actually help sustain a healthy quality of life. One study published in the *Journal of Epidemiology and Community Health* in 2016 showed that healthy people who postponed retirement by just one year had an 11 percent lower risk of dying. According to the study, even people with health problems who chose to postpone retirement lived longer. Waiting to retire also appears to also reduce the risk of Alzheimer's disease and dementia.

Your ability to keep working during your later years will pay dividends that extend beyond just your paycheck. Studies show that those who postponed retirement had a healthier financial portfolio. Financial security during retirement obviously makes life easier and healthier choices more available. Since financial pressure is one of the leading causes of stress in our country, avoiding any type of prolonged, chronic stressors will only improve your health.

On the other hand, retirement may be a healthier option if you have a very stressful job, do not like your job, or if you do not feel valued at work. In these cases, retirement might work to your advantage. If a job situation is detrimental to your mental health, if it is causing stress, or if it is not contributing to your own fulfillment of living your purpose, then retiring might be the answer for you.

To achieve optimal health during early retirement, it's important to create some other type of vocation. For some it is watching grandchildren or helping out family members. For others it might be growing a garden or crafting. Whatever the case, if you want to add life to your years in retirement, you will need to find some sort of fulfillment and purpose to fuel your life. You can serve your community by volunteering in the senior center, day care, or after-school program. Help out in your local city council office or development center. Of course, vacations, rest, and days where you do nothing can be important. However, eventually the retirees I have worked with usually receive fulfillment from serving their community. Establishing links to connect your life to others and find a place where you are needed can lend itself to maintaining a sense of purpose.

- Strength, mobility, and balance are essential to longevity and your quality of life.

- We are designed to move.

- Physical effort serves our muscles, bones, and joints.

- An active lifestyle is correlated with lower body weight, brighter moods, and a healthier stress response.

- It's never too late to find your soul mate of movements: walking, hiking, high interval intensity resistance training, swimming, weight lifting, tai chi, yoga, Pilates, dance, swimming, martial arts.

- If you work at a desk, stand up every 20 minutes.

- Remember a 3-minute walk every hour is enough to improve blood glucose levels.

- Every time you take or make a phone call, do it while walking or marching in place instead of sitting.

- Let your bed remind you to stretch. Here's how: Take 5 minutes to stretch in bed before getting up and stretch for 5 minutes in bed at night before you doze off.

- Practice incidental exercise. Park the car at the far end of the parking lot, take the stairs instead of the elevator, carry the groceries, put the water jug in the water dispenser—remember to squat and then lift, using your legs to protect your back. Yes, it all counts. Don't let anyone tell you different.

- Consider what it would it take to incorporate more exercise into your life. Would it mean going to sleep earlier, so you can get up an hour earlier?

1. How many days of the week do you exercise? (1 point per day, 7 points total)

2. How many days a week are you moving regularly? (1 point per day, 7 points total)

3. Are there any times during the week when you might use walking as your mode of transportation instead of a car, bus, or train? Y or N (1 point for yes)

4. Do you regularly practice one of the following forms of exercise: walking, hiking, high intensity interval resistance training, swimming, weight lifting, tai chi, yoga, Pilates, dance, swimming, martial arts, cycling? Y or N (1 point for each type of exercise)

5. Do you ever sit in a chair for more than one hour before getting up? Y or N (−1 point for yes)

6. Do you ever sit in a chair for more than two hours before getting up? Y or N (−2 points for yes)

7. Do you ever sit in a chair for more than three hours before getting up? Y or N (−3 points for yes)

8. Does your commute involve sitting in a car or train for more than thirty minutes? Y or N (−1 point for yes)

9. Does your commute involve sitting in a car or train for more than one hour? Y or N (−2 points for yes)

SCORE

0 points or less: You need to prioritize exercise and movement.

0 to 8 points: You're not a couch potato, but you could move more if you want to go the distance.

8 to 16 points: You're a pretty good mover and shaker.

16 or above: You're on track, super ager. Keep up the good work!

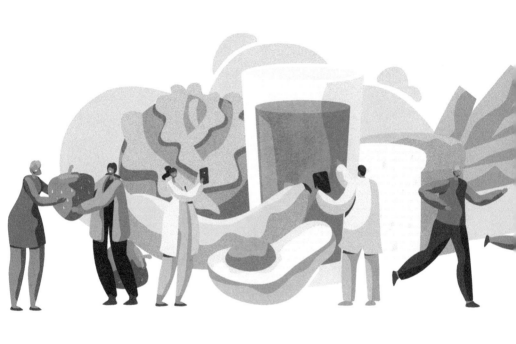

CHAPTER 3

Eat Real Food

O ver the last fifty years, the health industry has been constantly promoting new dietary fads. We have seen low-fat, high-carb, low-carb, high-protein, and high-fat diets, and everything in between. The commercial food industry then took advantage of the various health fads and presented a host of "food-like products"—convenient quick package foods—that claim to marry with these trending strategies.

When deciding on the optimal eating habits for your health, look at diets that have survived the test of time. Consider traditional food cultures that, along with culture and lifestyle patterns, have resulted in exceptional health and longevity.

FOOD FOR LIFE: THE MEDITERRANEAN DIET

The Mediterranean diet has stood the test of time. Study after study finds correlations between Mediterranean eating habits and heart health, optimal weight, and longevity.

The Mediterranean diet is based on plants. In fact, 90 percent of the Mediterranean diet is food that grew from the ground.

In 2013, researchers looked at 10,000 women on the Mediterranean diet and found that they were 40 percent more likely to live past age 70 without chronic illness, poor cognition, or mental problems. In general, research has demonstrated that those on the Mediterranean diet are less likely to die from heart attacks and stroke.

The Mediterranean diet is based on the food traditions of communities surrounding the Mediterranean Sea, especially Italy, Greece, and Crete. In fact, two of the five Blue Zones, Sardinia and Ikaria, are located on the Mediterranean Sea. It's important to take a look at the habits in those regions, while remembering that many of those traditions have been misrepresented in U.S. food culture. For example, in America, when we eat a double cheese pizza or mountainous bowl of spaghetti, we believe we're eating Italian food. However, this is not actually how people eat in Italy. If you order ravioli in Italy, you'll receive a plate with a few small pieces of pasta. To Italians, pasta is considered one course in a meal that includes salad, vegetables and, perhaps, some beans, meat, or fish.

Mediterranean cultures traditionally enjoy a daily, diverse array of vegetables, fruits, nuts, seeds, olives, legumes, beans, and whole grains. Fish is the main source of protein, with other meats eaten sparingly. The moderate consumption of wine is usually limited to one or two glasses.

The benefits of a Mediterranean diet are numerous. The diet is full of fiber, which slows digestion and reduces the dumping of sugar into the blood. Balancing blood sugar in this manner wards off mood swings, promotes energy throughout the day, and helps prevent diabetes.

There are virtually no processed foods in this diet. Not only is the consumption of toxic ingredients decreased, with high plant consumption, you have powerful antioxidants that sequester free radicals from toxins that would otherwise cause damage. The Mediterranean diet also helps decrease inflammation. Inflammation is the basis for most chronic diseases such as arthritis, heart disease, diabetes, Alzheimer's disease and dementia, and cancer. Finally, this diet is heart friendly, virtually a cholesterol-free diet. People who eat the Mediterranean diet tend to maintain a healthy weight throughout life without needing to go on special weight-loss diets. It is no wonder that this approach to eating well has stood the test of time.

CHOOSING QUALITY FOOD FOR LIFE

How is "quality food" defined? I define it as eating food in its natural state, food that is organic and unprocessed. This is food that has grown out of the earth, been plucked off a tree or bush, walked on the land, or was swimming in the sea. Whole foods have not been modified or taken apart. For example, root vegetables such as sweet potato, turnips, and beets grow in the earth. Asparagus, kale, broccoli, and artichokes have grown out of the earth. Lemons, figs, apples, and blueberries have been plucked off a tree or a bush. Grass-fed cows and pastured poultry have walked the land, and cod and sardines swam in the sea.

Conversely, a processed food product may contain ingredients that used to be a whole food but have since been cooked down, dehydrated, reconstituted, or sheared of some original ingredients, like the bran in wheat. Other examples are most commercial fruit or vegetable juices, which come from cooked and reconstituted produce, and items that sound like whole foods, such as rolled oats. Other obvious examples are packaged foods like chips, crackers, and fruit strips. They've passed through a factory or processing center and are delivered to you in a box or plastic container.

The epidemic of processed foods in America is a relatively new phenomenon. Industrial food is engineered to become tastier and then packaged to make it convenient. Consider the habit of picking up a box of cereal, for example. However, if longevity and good health are our goals, consumption of these nutrient-depleted foods must be greatly curbed.

When your great-great-grandmother prepared food, she had no alternative but to use mostly whole, unprocessed foods. She simply went to her garden or bought food from the local grocer, butcher, or fishmonger and cooked it. The food her family ate was grown or raised in her area and had been picked or slaughtered within days—or hours—of her purchase.

How Industrial Agriculture and the Food Industry Alter Food

Unless it comes from your garden or local organic farmer, it's likely that the food you buy at the grocery store has been altered even before it goes to a factory or packaging facility. In other words, industrial agricultural practices do not keep our food at the highest quality. Crops are heavily sprayed with pesticides and sometimes genetically modified. Our topsoil is depleted, and our animals are victims of the demands for mass production.

Processed foods have been broken down, then recombined with sugar, salt, and highly refined processed oils, as well as infused with dyes and chemicals. These chemicals are used as flavor enhancers, emulsifiers, dough conditioners, preservatives, and synthetic coloring. These processed items are put into a package with a marketing message—and a bucolic picture of lakes, fields, sunshine, or animals grazing to help you associate the product with a farm. In fact, much of what goes into such packages hasn't grown or walked around in a long time. That's one reason why they might put in all the additives. These interventions exist because the food industry relies on shipping food farther from where it's sourced and extending its shelf life for as long as possible.

The soy industry is a case study in understanding how a whole, nutritious food can be processed into an unhealthy product. Approximately 95 percent of the soy grown in America is genetically modified. In general, when Okinawans eat soy, it is in its pure form of edamame or a non-GMO organic firm tofu high in proteins and phytoestrogens. Genetically modified or processed soybeans found in vegetarian meat substitutes like "veggie" hot dogs, burgers, or "chicken" nuggets, etc. stress the immune system. The health benefits are lost and the processed soy may actually cause dangerous cellular and hormonal changes.

Shop for the Natural Version of All-Star Foods

Beans are a basic part of the Blue Zone and Mediterranean diets. People in the Blue Zones eat four times as many beans as anywhere else in the world. In Nicoya, black beans are eaten almost daily. Mediterranean eaters fill their diets with protein-rich lentils, garbanzo beans, and white beans. Beans contain protein and complex carbohydrates as well as many vitamins and minerals. In general, dried beans are unprocessed, safe, real foods. However, keep in mind that quality is important and eating organically will always trump conventionally grown beans.

Fish is another great source of protein found in the Mediterranean diet. In Sardinia, fish is eaten in small amounts, generally three to five ounces per meal at two or three meals per week. The fish consumed are sardines, anchovies, and cod. These are fish lower on the food chain and therefore have lower levels of contaminants such as mercury and polychlorinated biphenyls (PCBs).

Eggs eaten in the Mediterranean are mostly from small farms where the chickens are free to run around on the pasture instead of grown industrially in cages and given feed full of estrogen. Like fish, eggs are consumed in smaller quantities.

Mediterranean Foods

VEGETABLES	FRUITS	HERBS AND SPICES
Arugula/rocket	Apples	Anise
Beets	Apricots	Basil
Bok Choy	Cherries	Bay leaf
Broccoli	Clementines	Chilies
Broccolini	Dates	Cloves
Broccoli rabe	Figs	Cumin
Brussels sprouts	Grapefruit	Fennel
Cabbage	Grapes	Garlic
Carrots	Lemons	Lavender
Cauliflower	Melons	Marjoram
Celery	Nectarines	Mint
Collard greens	Olives	Oregano
Eggplant	Oranges	Parsley
Fennel	Peaches	Pepper
Garden cress	Pears	Pul biber (Aleppo pepper)
Horseradish	Pomegranates	Rosemary
Kale	Pumpkin	Sage
Kohlrabi	Strawberries	Tarragon
Komatsuna	Tangerines	Thyme
Leeks	Tomatoes	Turmeric
Lettuce		Za'atar
Mâche		
Mizuna		
Mustard greens		
Napa (Chinese) cabbage		
Okra		
Onion		
Peppers		
Radishes		
Rutabaga		
Scallions		
Shallots		
Spinach		
Squash		
Sweet potatoes		
Tatsoi		
Turnip		
Zucchini		

LEGUMES, BEANS	BEANS, NUTS, SEEDS	OIL, FAT
Cannellini	Almonds	Olive oil
Chickpeas	Brazil nuts	Avocado
Fava beans	Cashews	Grass-fed cow butter
Green peas	Chia	
Lentils	Flax	
Split peas	Pine nuts	
	Pistachios	
	Pumpkin	
	Sesame	
	Sunflower	
	Walnuts	

DAIRY	EGGS, FISH, MEAT	GRAINS
Brie	Chicken eggs	Amaranth
Chèvre	Duck eggs	Barley
Feta	Quail eggs	Brown rice
Halloumi	Cod	Buckwheat
Manchego	Flounder	Bulgur
Parmigiano-Reggiano	Mackerel	Farro
Pecorino	Salmon	Freekeh
Ricotta	Sardines	Millet
Greek yogurt	Sea bass	Polenta
(watch this category if you are lactose intolerant)	Tuna	Quinoa
	Yellowtail	Teff
	Beef	Wheat berries
	Goat	
	Lamb	

They are never a main dish and are always a side dish, most people consuming only two to four eggs per week. In the United States, estrogen is placed in the chicken feed in order to make the chicken lay eggs faster and in larger numbers. This is great for the egg industry, but not very good for our human bodies. Our bodies process these estrogens and that affects fertility in a negative way. These exogenous estrogens—or what the scientific community calls "synthetic xenoestrogens"—are associated with diabetes, obesity, fibroids, and infertility.

Cow's milk is another food we have to be wary of in the Standard American Diet (SAD). Almost 60 percent of Americans are lactose intolerant, where the lactose in milk causes digestive upset. However, that's not all! What most don't realize is the immune system goes into overdrive, weakening the body. In the Mediterranean diet, most milk is from goat or sheep milk. In general goat and sheep milk are hypoallergenic. The goat milk may contain lactose, but it also contains lactase, an enzyme that helps you break down lactose. People living and eating in the Mediterranean do not experience the same kind of digestive disorders that many Americans are experiencing.

Overall, meat, including fish and animal products such as milk and eggs, are eaten sparingly, less than 10 percent in both the Mediterranean diet and in the Blue Zones in general. Plants, on the other hand make up almost 95 percent of the diet! It is very important that the 95 percent is made up of mostly vegetarian forms of protein like beans, seeds, and nuts along with a plethora of vegetables. I mention this because I find that some of my patients consume a diet full of bread, rice, and pasta. In a sense, you could say they are still following a plant-based, vegetarian diet. But the Mediterranean diet is the model diet that gives all the benefits. Again, quality and quantity matter.

To Drink or Not to Drink? Is That the Question?

It's important to approach alcohol carefully. Alcohol consumption has been associated with several types of cancer, especially breast cancer. However, the Mediterranean diet, which is plant rich and therefore nutrient dense with a high antioxidant status, also generally incorporates some wine. One or two drinks of high-quality, low-pesticide wine is generally considered safe and may even contribute to improved heart health.

Red wine is unique in that it contains a component called resveratrol, which is found in the skin of red wine grapes. Resveratrol may be the key to why red wine, if consumed in moderation—no more than two glasses per day—may add to your life. Please note that, if you have trouble limiting your consumption of alcohol, the benefits of wine do not outweigh the detrimental effects of consuming too much.

Longevity Foods

Red wine (one to two glasses): This contains antioxidants like resveratrol which promote longevity.

Olive oil: Ikarians eat about six tablespoons of a high-flavanol olive oil per day, which can cut the risk of dying in half.

Seeds: These mini power foods contain all the food groups and more: protein, fat, complex carbohydrates, fiber, vitamins, minerals, and antioxidants.

Leafy green vegetables: Spinach, kale, collards, chard, beet tops, and turnip tops are full of antioxidants that promote longevity.

FROM THE HEART

Cardiovascular disease remains the leading cause of death in the United States. According to the latest statistics from the American Heart Association, 46 percent of American adults have hypertension. Eating processed food; forgoing exercise; smoking; having high blood pressure; and suffering from obesity, lack of sleep, and stress are all precursors to heart attack or stroke. These precursors are correctable through simple lifestyle changes.

Your first ally may be, once again, the Mediterranean diet. High in healthy fats and antioxidants and low in inflammatory fats and processed foods, this dietary style is linked with stronger cardiovascular health, cleaner arteries, and reduced risk of strokes.

Here are some heart-healthy tips at a glance:

- Eat fish that contain omega-3 fatty acids

- Eat other good fats like avocado, nuts, and seeds

- Drink one glass of high-quality red wine per day (optional) and limit other alcohol

- Exercise your heart three to six days a week

- Manage your stress

- Choose natural sea salt over refined, processed salt—and still sprinkle lightly

- Cut out refined sugar

- Remove bad fats from your diet such as canola or vegetable oil or anything with trans fats

- If you smoke, keep quitting until you stop for good

EATING FOR THE BRAIN: THE MIND DIET

Dementia rates in the United States and industrialized world are higher than in parts of the world that have yet to modernize away from their traditional eating habits. One reason may be the industrialization of our food supply, which creates a nutritional deficit coupled with additional toxins that our bodies need to process.

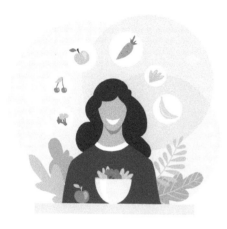

Thank goodness there is much we can do to preserve our brain health. Enter the MIND diet. This protocol, the Mediterranean-DASH Intervention for Neurodegenerative Delay, will sound very much like the Mediterranean diet. It pairs that basic plant-based, whole-foods approach with some lessons from the DASH diet, which is a very effective protocol for combating hypertension. The DASH diet promotes getting high fiber from fruit, vegetable, whole grains, beans, and nuts. Plus, it includes lean meats like protein and fish. On the DASH diet, fat was generally discouraged, but with the MIND diet, we look for where the Mediterranean and DASH diet meet on common ground.

Research finds that pairing these approaches points to several foods that are particularly helpful for brain health, especially in those who are already experiencing symptoms of cognitive decline. For example, berries—more than other fruits—appear to improve both heart and brain health. This could be due to the high antioxidant and flavonol content in berries, which strengthens the arteries and therefore increases blood supply to the heart and the brain.

MIND Foods to Eat:

1. Berries: strawberries, blueberries, cranberries, goji berries, black raspberries, mulberries, etc.

2. Green leafy vegetables

3. Vegetables

4. Nuts

5. Olive oil

6. Beans

7. Fish

8. Poultry

9. Whole grains

10. Wine

Foods to Avoid on the MIND Diet:

1. Butter (unless grass-fed, see below)

2. Cheese

3. Red meat

4. Fried foods

5. Refined, bleached flour and foods made from processed flour

Healthy Fat

The brain cell membranes are made up of fatty tissue that benefits from healthy fats, such as those found in avocado, nuts, seeds, olives, and certain fish. Let's take a closer look:

Coconut oil: This oil contains keto bodies that the brain can accept and use as fuel without also requiring insulin. This makes coconut oil an especially strong ally for diabetics and others with blood sugar issues. In addition to protecting the brain, it's associated with improving cognitive function among people with Alzheimer's disease, boosting liver health, and promoting weight loss.

Grass-fed butter: Butter from grass-fed cattle—meaning cows raised on their natural diet of grass—has many benefits over commercial butter. It contains the beneficial omega-6 oil called conjugated linoleic acid (CLA) which can neutralize chronic inflammation. Grass-fed butter is also more nutritious than the butter made from cows that feed on grains, soy, corn, and apple core. Much of their feed tends to have GMO ingredients which will get into the butter.

Cold-water fish: Eating cold-water fish and supplementing with fish oils provides high levels of omega-3 fatty acids. Omega-3 fatty acids used to be present in the American diet. However, they have been bred out of vegetables in order to help with extending their shelf lives. Fat tends to go rancid quickly, so if it is removed from a vegetable, that plant will appear fresh on the shelf longer. Fish oils help build excellent brain cell membranes and quell inflammation in the brain. Krill oil might be a particularly powerful brain ally as it contains phospholipids that help the nervous system assimilate omega-3 fatty acids. However, it is important to note that krill does not have nearly the amount of omega-3s that other fish oil does, so supplementing with both might be best.

YOUR BRAIN LOVES A CHALLENGE

One of the best ways to love your brain is to challenge it. The old "use it or lose it" adage definitely applies here, as under-utilized brain cells tend to fizzle out over time. Some believe that because they are thinking all day, they're using their brain. However, it's easy to fall into familiar mental habits. What you want to do instead is stimulate your brain with a diverse range of tasks, including fresh challenges that get the cognitive gears turning. When you give your brain novel experiences, such as using your hands and body in unusual ways, engaging in unexpected conversations, and looking for ways to think differently, you encourage neuroplasticity. Neuroplasticity is the ability of the brain to form new synaptic connections, a process that protects brain cells and encourages the growth of new brain tissue.

Here are some easy ways to stimulate or "stretch" your brain throughout the day:

- Learn a new physical skill or study a new language or subject.

- Take a different route home, whether driving or walking.

- Keep up with technology

- Try Scrabble, Sudoku, word searches, or crossword puzzles.
- Check out a dance class like Zumba or learn to waltz or tango.
- Strike up more conversations.
- Study the life story of a world leader, celebrity, or business mogul of interest to you.
- Read a different section of the newspaper.
- Break your standard reading routine and pick up a newspaper or magazine you've never read before.
- Read poetry or a novel, especially if you usually read non-fiction—or vice versa.
- Listen to a radio station you would normally skip past—especially if it features opinions you disagree with.
- Use scissors or a fork with your nondominant hand from time to time.
- Use one of your six senses combined with a motor skill. For example, listen to music while painting.

MICROBIOME BASICS

What Is the Microbiome?

Another important concept related to food, brain health, and longevity is the microbiome. The microbiome consists of all the bacteria, yeasts, protozoa, and viruses located mostly in our gut. The gut is a thirty-foot-long tube that extends from our mouths

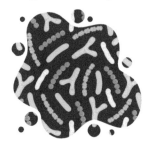 to our anus. Most of the microbiome lives there, but it also covers skin and hair and may even follow us around, not unlike Pig-Pen in the *Peanuts* comic strip. The microbiome weighs anywhere from one to five pounds per person.

What Does It Mean for Health?

Mostly through a very large study called the Human Genome Project, scientists found some very important information to influence our health in a positive way. First, we had always known the brain instructs our digestive tract through the vagus nerve. However, never did we understand that communication between the gut and the brain is bidirectional, meaning the digestive tract also tells the brain what to do. In fact, the gut is known as "the second brain." On some level, we have already intuitively had this understanding as there are so many idioms that express this concept: "Listen to your gut," "I had a gut feeling," "I have butterflies in my stomach," etc.

Previously, the prevailing idea was that only the brain had neurotransmitters. In fact, the brain's nervous system, or the central nervous system, and the gut's nervous system, or enteric nervous system, each harbor the same number of neurotransmitters. Neurotransmitters are important for affecting behaviors such as appetite, sleep, fear, and mood. A particularly mind-blowing finding has been that 90 percent of the body's serotonin—the "feel-good" hormone—is found in the gut. When treating a patient, I like to make sure that the gut and brain are communicating and functioning harmoniously with each other. My husband likes the expression "happy wife, happy life." Similarly, you could say, "happy gut, happy life." The gut and brain are better versions of themselves when they have a good marriage with lots of sharing and communication.

Scientists have also discovered that good levels of neurotransmitters are correlated with a rich, diverse supply of friendly bacteria. That's right. Despite the amount of antibacterial soap and hand sanitizer we use in the United States, we are not sterile and that's great. In fact, we need a vast array of friendly bacteria for optimal health. High levels of good bacteria in your microbiota regulate your immune system and can help you ward off and fight infections such as food poisoning, urinary tract and bladder infections, vaginitis, and even your regular cold and flu. A weak microbiota—one featuring a low diversity of bacteria and low levels of the most beneficial organisms—can predispose you to allergies, autoimmune conditions, and numerous other health issues. Your digestive health greatly relies on the probiotics in your microbiota. It helps you make vitamin K, which is important for blood clotting, calcium levels in your blood, and bone metabolism. Probiotics can regulate bowel movements and support a healthy gut overall.

Where Does a Strong Microbiome Come From?
Human beings get their original microbiome from their parents. As babies pass through the vaginal canal, they pick up plenty of healthy bacteria from the mother. The baby will swallow some bacteria, then growth factors in the mother's milk help the bacteria colonize in baby's gut. This suggests that naturally birthed and breastfed babies are the strongest babies. And, please don't get me wrong, ALL birth is good. Mothers might plan for and idealize a natural, vaginal birth, but, ultimately, a cesarean birth may be required. Regardless of how you were born and whether or not you were breastfed, the health and diversity of your microbiota should and can be cultivated and optimized throughout your life.

Many circumstances can affect your gut flora. Studies demonstrate that siblings often share microbiome composition, with the youngest sibling having the most diverse microbiota. In twin studies, the obese twin has a less diverse microbiome than the lean twin. Other studies show that trauma and health challenges can also affect the microbiome. We know that people with PTSD and autism have different microbiota makeups than people without those conditions. Autoimmune diseases such as multiple sclerosis, rheumatoid arthritis, and fibromyalgia are also associated with microbiomes that lack diversity.

How to Protect Your Gut Microbiome

Many factors support an optimal microbiota. Think of the lining of your intestine as coveted real estate with thousands of varieties of yeast, parasites, bacteria, and protozoans all competing to acquire property. The lifestyle choices we make, the toxic exposures, and what we eat deters or promotes the growth and proliferation of friendly bacteria. When the friendly bacteria are robust, they will crowd out less-helpful organisms. For example, high levels of good bacteria keep yeast levels within a healthy range.

The first step you can take toward a powerful microbiota is to clean up the environment in your body. Try to prevent pesticides, false hormones, and antibiotics from entering your body. Conventional foods and meats can contain all three of these harmful chemicals. Other substances to avoid are sugar, high-fructose corn syrup and artificial sweeteners, trans fats, and hydrogenated fats. Processed foods in general—those that come in a box or plastic container—generally contain these unwanted additives. Eating a diet of organically grown food is a critical step in maintaining a clean, gut-friendly inner landscape.

That overlaps with the next step, which is to feed your bacterial allies. That involves consuming prebiotics, foods that specifically nourish good bacteria. Remember that they're living creatures and need to eat like everybody else. It turns out that the good guys of the bacterial world thrive on fiber-rich, fresh produce. Look for "shooting" greens such as asparagus, leeks, scallions, and ramps (garlic spears). Garlic and onions will also provide prebiotics. Look for fermented foods such as sauerkraut, kimchi, miso, and kefir water or kefir, preferably from coconut milk or almond milk or cow's milk if you tolerate dairy well. Fiber found in legumes, nuts, seeds, and good fats such as coconut and olive oil all promote the growth of a strong microbiome.

The great news is the diets that promote longevity—the diets eaten in the Blue Zones, the Mediterranean diet, and the MIND diet—are all congruent with a diet that would cultivate a rich microbiome. So all paths lead to the same nutritional super-highway, and it is lined with fresh unprocessed whole foods, mostly made up of fiber-rich plants.

WHEN TO SUPPLEMENT

My patients are sometimes resistant to taking supplements. They want to get all their nutrients from food. Although noble in aspiration, and perhaps achievable during our great-great-grandmother's time, it can be difficult to reach this goal now, particularly if you're already recovering from illness or health setbacks. In my family, we try to consume a balanced, nutrient-dense diet by shopping at our local health food store, growing our own fresh herbs and spices, and getting our food through a community-shared agriculture (CSA) or directly from the farmer. We cook and prepare food for ourselves daily. And, yet, we also supplement.

Supplements should be just that—nutrients to supplement our diets. We need to supplement because industrial agriculture has depleted the diverse mineral content of our topsoil and therefore our food supply.

When supplementing for the family, there are certain foundational supplements I think are important to ward off disease, help you live a wonderful quality of life, replenish nutrients missing from the diet, and extend your life.

Probiotics: help promote colonization and growth of the microbiome

Vitamin D$_3$: the large majority of the population is extremely deficient. While blood work might show the range of normal to be above 30 ng/m (nanograms per milliliter), most are below 30. Those that have reached 30 have good bone protection. However, people who increase their vitamin D status to the 50 to 100 range have help in protecting themselves from heart disease, diabetes, hip fractures, colds and flus, and perhaps even cancer.

Fish oil: Another major deficiency in humans is omega-3 fatty acids. These oils sequester inflammation. Inflammation might be the ultimate cause of all aging and chronic disease, but we know that fish oils contribute to what I like to think of as oiling and lubing the inside of your body. Without these oils incorporated into your body, your tissues become dry and hard. Omega-3 oils from fish oils are absorbed into the brain cell wall, making the cell more plastic and able to bend and conform as needed, allowing brain cells to dump out garbage, intake nutrition, and communicate cell to cell. Omega-3s incorporated into blood vessels help make the artery stretchy and compliant instead of hard and brittle, which might contribute to poor artery health.

Multivitamins: Industrial agriculture and poor-quality topsoil, coupled with the most toxic environment that the human body has ever had to deal with, makes for poor nutritional status with an increased nutritional demand. Many of my patients report feeling more energy and clarity after they begin taking a multivitamin.

Magnesium: Again, due to industrial agriculture, our soil has become depleted of minerals. Magnesium is the number one human mineral deficiency. By replenishing your magnesium status, you might be able to relax, literally. Magnesium allows you to relax blood vessels, leading to lower pressure, which helps you handle stress and can help with insomnia. This mineral also seems to help with constipation by relaxing your bowels. Many people are able to relieve chronic tension headaches just by adding magnesium supplementation.

These are the supplements that promote longevity, prevent cognitive decline, and provide multiple support structures, giving you more bang for your buck.

Resveratrol: Resveratrol is a phytonutrient called a polyphenol, not unlike an antioxidant. It is believed that plants develop polyphenols to ward off fungi and bacteria as they grow. You can find resveratrol in the skin of grapes, red wine, berries, and from the Japanese plant called *Polygonum cuspidatum*, also known as Japanese knotweed. In each one of our cells we have a mitochondrion, which is considered to be the engine or powerhouse of the cell. It is what cranks out energy. The trillions of mitochondria produce fuel that results in the cumulative energy that we use and feel.

As we age, some of the mitochondria age and are rendered useless. Resveratrol recycles and renews our mitochondria. It helps us produce energy again like we did when we were younger. A truly antiaging supplement and prolonger of life, resveratrol appears to turn on genes that defend against disease. Resveratrol can also support blood glucose levels, and it may help improve lean body mass in older adults. It appears to support lipid levels and blood pressure already in a normal range. And finally, there is some preliminary research showing resveratrol may help with preserving an aging brain.

Oligo proanthocyanidins (OPCs): OPCs are an extremely strong phenols and antioxidants that are much stronger than vitamin E and vitamin C. You can find them in seeds, seed coats, and skins of purple-pigmented foods such as berries and grapes as well as French maritime pine trees. OPCs powerfully remove inflammation from our bodies. They can help normalize blood pressure, strengthen blood vessel walls, and give support with allergies and skin health.

Curcumin from turmeric: Turmeric and its curcumins are arguably the strongest natural anti-inflammatory out there. Turmeric is the root of the *Curcuma longa* plant. It looks similar to ginger, yet when you cut it open it is a bright yellow, almost orange color. This pigment is the constituent in turmeric called curcumin. Curcumin makes up about 2 or 3 percent of the turmeric root, yet this is what is mostly responsible for the benefits you receive when taking turmeric. You can take both turmeric and curcumin as supplements. In general, I encourage people to cook with turmeric and take curcumin as a supplement.

In concert with its anti-inflammatory properties, curcumin supports the body's fight against age-related chronic disease such as cardiovascular disease, cognitive decline and Alzheimer's disease, osteoarthritis, and rheumatoid arthritis. It may also lower your risk for cancer. My patients suffering from arthritis seem to benefit the most from curcumin supplementation. The most dramatic patient testimonial came from a patient of mine who was suffering with arthritis in her hands for a year. Two days after taking the curcumin supplement I supplied to her, the pain disappeared.

Cocoa: By cocoa, we mean high-flavanol cocoa that you can get from your health food store and take as a supplement or mix into your smoothies. Do not mistake this for quick-mix grocery store packets that have chemicals, sugar, and cholesterol added. Cocoa appears to contribute to longevity by strengthening blood vessels and improving circulation, among other benefits. Cocoa crosses the blood-brain barrier and can enhance brain function and mood.

The Kuna people live on small islands off the coast of Panama. Here, high-flavanol cocoa grows in abundance, and the Kuna drink it daily. The Kuna appear to have lower blood pressure and live longer than other Panamanians. Many factors are responsible for the lower incidences of heart attacks, strokes, diabetes, and cancer among the Kunas. But it is important to note that cocoa might play a significant role in the Kuna achieving this.

Green tea: One of the most researched and widely consumed plants out there, green tea, from the *Camellia sinensis* plant, shines as a panacea. It can help prevent dangerous cellular changes, increase a slow metabolism, support cardiovascular health, normalize blood fats, and regulate blood sugar. Plus, it is a powerful antioxidant, has anti-inflammatory properties, and is antimicrobial.

Melatonin: As we get older, our melatonin levels—hormones that help us fall asleep and stay asleep—become depleted. A melatonin supplement is a very safe way of replenishing your melatonin levels. Getting sleep is very important for the body to heal, restore, and prevent cognitive decline.

Collagen: Once we hit our second decade of life, we lose about 1 percent of collagen per year. The word collagen comes from the Greek word *kolla*, meaning glue. Think of collagen as the glue that holds us together. Collagen loss is associated with sagging skin, wrinkles, and poor joint health because collagen makes up the cartilage in our joints.

Whey: A protein powder, whey can help us keep our muscle as we get older. Whey also has a blood-pressure-lowering effect. However, if you have dairy intolerance, you might do better with a plant-based protein powder.

Acetyl-L-Carnitine: This amino acid, in combination with alpha lipoic acid, can help maintain nerve and brain function as well as glucose metabolism.

DROP THE FORK A LITTLE SOONER

In my private practice, many patients come to me for weight management. Indeed, obesity is an epidemic in the United States. It can be very complicated: food intolerance, GMOs, hormones, stress, emotional eating, insomnia, and poor nutritional status—whether overfed or undernourished—all play a role. Therefore, saying something like "eat less and exercise more" is often ineffectual and may even be detrimental to some people. Yet, on the other hand, a lot of pounds could be dropped simply by eating smaller portions. In America, our culture states, "eat until you are full." In Okinawa, the elders say, "eat until you are no longer hungry."

However, weight management is not the only reason an elder Okinawan might say *hara hachi bu* before a meal, which roughly translates to "belly eight parts full." It's the practice of eating until you are 80 percent full, and Okinawans often say it before a meal as a reminder. Longevity studies show that this type of light eating leads to stronger digestion and a longer, healthier, and better quality of life. Okinawans have one of the lowest rates of illness from heart disease, cancer, and stroke, with a longer life expectancy than most people in the world.

HOW TO KNOW YOU ARE 80 PERCENT FULL:

Eat slowly. It takes 20 minutes for your stomach to digest food and send a signal to the brain that it is filling up. If you scarf down your plate in 10 minutes, you might not have realized that you've already passed the point of contentment.

Practice mindful eating. In addition to eating slowly, it's important to eat without distraction. I encourage you not to read, watch TV, or look at your smartphone. Put the fork down between bites. If you are eating with company, quiet conversation can slow down the pace.

Chew your food very thoroughly, for several seconds. Relax and enjoy your meal. This slow pace is critical for allowing your body to register what you're eating so it can generate the appropriate enzymes for breaking down and extracting nutrients from that particular type of food. Without this process, you can end up with poorly digested food moving through your digestive system. This can promote inflammation in addition to depriving you of nutrients.

Many Americans of a certain age were raised with the idea that eating everything on their plate was a form of good behavior. In a school where my husband taught, they practiced the "Happy Plate." A happy plate was an empty plate, and the child who finished his food was verbally rewarded. This practice seems outdated—and possibly dangerous—given what we know now. For one thing, it teaches a child to keep eating regardless of the cues they're getting from their body. If you are going for longevity and masterful aging, the new happy plate may have some food left on it.

- The Mediterranean diet is nutrient dense and rich in fiber.

- It can help maintain a healthy weight, balance blood sugar, provide fiber, decrease and eliminate toxins, decrease inflammation, and support the heart and brain.

- The diet consists of vegetables, fruits, nuts, seeds, olives, olive oil, legumes, beans, whole grains, fish, and some meat.

- A healthy microbiome is associated with good digestion, a stronger immune system, and a healthier brain, among others.

- A vibrant microbiome is cultivated and protected by eating a high-fiber, organic diet with lots of vegetables and as little sugar and processed food as possible.

- Start shopping at farmers' markets and look for a community-supported agriculture (CSA) service that delivers food from local farms.

- Remove heavily processed, inflammatory commercial oils such as corn, soy, vegetable, canola, and shortening from your kitchen.

- Replace them with unprocessed extra-virgin olive oil, coconut oil, grass-fed butter, or ghee, as well as grapeseed and avocado oil for higher heat.

- You can never have too many vegetables. Where can you add vegetables throughout each meal?

- Try a new seafood recipe and start bringing more of these healthy fats and proteins into your life.

- Add beans. The longest-living people in the world eat beans.

- If eating beans causes a gassy belly, you may not have the enzymes and gut flora necessary to digest them. For most of us—given there are no other underlying digestive issues—consuming just one teaspoonful of beans for a few days in a row can help your body create those enzymes.

- Try different nut or seed butters. In the morning, you can add sunflowers, walnuts, or pumpkin seeds to your cereal, porridge, or smoothie. Have a handful as a snack with a piece of fruit.

- Save sugar for only very special occasions.

- I recommend always supplementing. Basics are a multivitamin, fish oil or DHA from algae, probiotic, and vitamin D. If you get a boost of energy or a feeling of well-being, stick with that supplement.

- Practice eating mindfully. Tune into your body to notice when you are 80 percent full.

1. How often do you eat vegetables per week? (1 point per day of the week)

2. How many servings of vegetables do you get in a day? (1 point per serving in a day)

3. How many days of the week do you have a plant-based protein like legumes or beans? (1 point per day of the week)

4. Do you have fish or eggs a few times per week? Y or N (2 points for yes)

5. Do you have seeds or nuts a few times per week? Y or N (3 points for yes)

6. Do you shop at farmers' markets, health food stores, or belong to a CSA? Y or N (2 points for yes, –2 points for no)

7. Do you shop organic? Y or N (2 points for yes, –2 points for no)

8. Do you shop for local produce? Y or N (2 points for yes)

9. Do you have extra-virgin olive oil, coconut oil, avocado oil daily or regularly? Y or N (2 points for yes)

10. Do you chew your food completely—about 32 chews per bite? Y or N (2 points for yes)

11. Do you cook with unhealthy oils (corn, vegetable, soy, shortening, lard) or eat at restaurants weekly where they most likely do not use healthy oils? (–1 point for every day you eat out or for unhealthy oils in your kitchen)

12. Do you eat sugar daily or more than four times per week? Y or N (–4 points for yes)

13. Do you eat products made from refined, processed flour daily? Y or N (–7 points for yes)

14. Do you eat products from refined, processed flour more than 3 times per week? (–3 points for yes)

SCORE

8 points or less: Becoming a masterful ager will definitely require some work on your nutrition.

8 to 12 points: You have some healthy habits but your nutrition could use some fine-tuning.

12 to 20 points: Impressive!

20 or above: Bon appétit, super ager. Keep up the good work!

CHAPTER 4

Connect

Research has shown us that relationships, socialization, and spiritual support go hand in hand with longevity and super aging. Those with meaningful relationships and time to socialize tend to live longer and are happier. In fact, according to a review of 148 studies containing over 300,000 study participants, it was determined that social isolation is a major risk factor for early mortality, and perhaps even a greater risk factor than obesity, smoking, and high blood pressure. Conversely, participating in an environment where socialization is promoted and cultivated—like in a church community—can add up to 14 more years to a person's life. Socialization might increase your chance of longevity by 50 percent. If you want to be a master ager, you will need to get out and socialize. For some of you, this might be a welcome invitation, but for others who are shy, socialization might be a super-aging skill that you will need to acquire. The good news is, you can do it. A phrase from my Louise L. Hay affirmation calendar reads, "I bring a joyful playmate into my life, and we have so much fun." Set the intention to find that one joyful playmate and start there.

RELATIONSHIPS

I have often heard the statement "family is everything" tossed around. I acknowledge that the phrase sounds trite. However, I have since come to realize that family can refer to all the people that you surround yourself with every day. Relationships and how we treat each other, how we respond to that treatment, and what we learn from those interactions form the basis of how we cope with stress, heal, and find joy and purpose in our day.

If abuse has ever been part of your life, you will need to create new, enriching relationships to foster healing and wholeness. With my patients, I have found that physical healing and vitality are often possible only after the patient addresses fundamental relationships, particularly with their parents. On the other hand, if you get along with your family—blood relatives or otherwise—continue making memories and nurturing your relationships. This is also a vehicle by which to put more life in your years.

For some, family and loved ones can be the reason for living and they act as a powerful reference point when making life choices. As a mother, I've also experienced the challenges of family life. In fact, having five children hasn't always helped me further my health goals. There have even been times when motherhood seemed like an excuse not to take care of myself. I would catch myself saying, I have five children so:

- I cannot exercise today.

- Who has time for meal prep?

- I don't have time to market my business.

- I will never get the opportunity to go on a vacation.

However, I eventually took a hard look at my narratives—and how I was feeling in my body. Then I asked myself, "What am I teaching my children when I forget self-care or when I don't exercise?" Could I be teaching them that they are the reason I don't take care of myself? Could I be teaching them that motherhood means sacrificing your physical health and emotional well-being and only serving others? Is that how I would want them to feel when and if they become mothers? No, it wasn't. I wanted them to feel empowered—and I wanted to set the right example. Now my children have become my reason. Here are my new thoughts:

- I will exercise today to set an example for my five daughters.

- I make time for meal prep to make sure we eat healthy foods to stave off colds and flus, to strengthen us, to live with energy, and to empower us.

- I will market my business and earn money and have leftover money to give to my girls so that I may take them to a great restaurant, pay for soccer lessons, travel the world with them, and make more memories.

- I go on vacation to get me time and to rejuvenate and recharge. Or, I take my family on vacation so we can experience new adventures together.

Do you see the difference? Now I am empowered instead of burdened. And life sounds more joyful and exciting, definitely one worth living for a long, long time.

Relationships bring meaningful interaction, service, rapport, connectedness, and love. A centenarian does not reach one hundred in isolation. When centenarians have long-term spouses, they support and grow together. A widowed centenarian often has a son, daughter, or a grandchild who looks after them and that they in turn nurture. Centenarians, in their later lives, have an evolved role, often acting as the "wise elder" to whom adult children come for advice and support.

Many grandparents enjoy their grandchildren without the burden of responsibility. With grandparents comes more love for the grandchildren as well as another voice of encouragement. They may also be an important keeper of cultural traditions for the younger generation. This focus on family, support, culture, and connectedness is a system that promotes longevity.

Love Rules

In an interview conducted with Dr. Brené Brown, a research professor at the University of Houston known for her studies on vulnerability, shame, and social connection, she stated, "A deep sense of love and belonging is an irresistible need of all people. We are biologically, cognitively, physically, and spiritually wired to love, to be loved, and to belong. When those needs are not met, we don't function as we were meant to. We break. We fall apart. We numb. We ache. We hurt others. We get sick." It is important to express and cultivate love in our relationships.

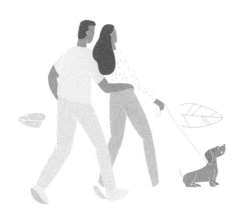

Sometimes in our busy lives we are comfortable with our family members knowing we love them, but we don't take time to verbally or physically express it. If you want to add years to your life, and subsequently your loved ones' lives, you might consider this. Cuddle time is a great way to do this. Cuddle your children, cuddle your partner, cuddle yourself. Just a few minutes on the couch can help you attain your cuddle quota. Have you heard of the six-second kiss?

The six-second kiss was first suggested by Dr. John Gottman, a relationship researcher. Six seconds is enough time for a couple to experience the intimacy and love they have between them. A peck on the cheek— though still a loving gesture—is not enough time to release oxytocin, also known as the "love" hormone that can cultivate loving bonds between people. This is the same hormone that gets released when a mother breastfeeds her child. Six seconds is all it takes to ensure love rules.

The Family That Eats Together Thrives Together

I cannot overstate how important communal meals are. Research demonstrates that eating meals together makes for better family bonds. By having meals together, family members get a fundamental lesson on how to eat well and subsequently choose to eat healthier as a result. Eating together also often helps the family's financial bottom line. People who eat family meals also suffer much less stress and depression.

Family meals support a secure foundation. This ritualized time together leaves children with an education on how to connect and speak with others. My husband calls it "home training." Home training helps us feel confident when we go out into the world; we feel more secure in how to act and speak to other people, making for better and more relationships. In Dan Buettner's *National Geographic* cover story, "The Secrets of a Long Life," there is a beautiful picture of centenarian Giovanni Sannai sitting at the head of a long oblong table of 18 family members in Sardinia, Italy (one of the Blue Zones). If you want to live past 100, this is dining at its best.

Healthy vs. Unhealthy Relationships

If you want to live a long and healthy life, relationships should promote your personal development and growth. Toxic relationships can be defined as relationships that bring you down and do not promote your growth. Some people in life have negative attitudes. They complain, gossip about others, put you down, and can be jealous of your relationships with other people. Sometimes the specific combination of you and the other person has you spending more time in an argument or leaves you both feeling badly. Research done at UCLA showed that social stressors in the form of conflict increased inflammation in the body. Excess inflammation accelerates aging. These are not the types of relationships you want to cultivate, especially if you are trying to master aging.

Jim Rohn said it best when he said you are the average of the five people you spend time around the most. If you look at the five people you spend the most time around, and you are not feeling excited and inspired and totally in love, you might consider swapping a really negative friend for a super supportive, very kind, and positive person. Now, I understand that sometimes we can't swap people out. If you've been living with a cousin you find negative, perhaps you can move out, and then see them only at family gatherings. However, if it is your mom or someone you married, consider therapy or marriage counseling. You might need outside help to give you feedback and the tools you need to cope and transform the relationship. Sometimes working on yourself is all you need, and the negative person might not want to be around you any longer.

COMMUNITY

We have discussed the importance of individual relationships and family ties. But understand that these individual relationships often happen within the context of a community or tribe.

Tribes

It is human nature to form groups or squads. This is because it is ingrained in our way of being to move and live in tribes. Tribes are united by commonalities, interests, culture, religion, and in some tribes, blood ties. There is usually a dialect or distinct way of speaking and sometimes a leader. There are rituals, commitments, and expectations that keep us involved; this structure is good for humans who do well on great habits. In the days before cell phones and electricity and even houses and apartments, people lived within their tribe. If they were going to move a few miles away, that was a tribal decision, and all people moved together, because isolation from the tribe equaled death. We needed to stay in our tribes in order to survive.

Now, because of modern technology, you do not have to move with your tribe. Modern living has made it so that you can be as independent as you would like. In fact, you do not even have to see anyone in person to have a social meeting or business transaction. However, in order to master aging and have a long vibrant life, we must stay connected. Existing within a community helps us thrive, not just survive. In modern culture, feeling part of a tribe or community allows us to meet our basic needs of security, reassurance, kindness, connection, and care.

A sense of belonging is important for our mental health and happiness, and—as I mentioned earlier—centenarians do not become centenarians in isolation. Communities can also give us purpose. Since we have commonalities, we feel like we belong. It can also give us a sense of fulfillment and accomplishment if we have skills or experience that we can contribute for the betterment of happiness of all. I encourage you to look for ways to volunteer or engage with your immediate neighborhood or wider community.

A community can also be a form of constructive entertainment. Social connections can bring out our passion and excitement about a hobby or interest. When we are learning, we are growing, which is an excellent message to send to the body as a signal to thrive. Like a simple houseplant, if the plant is not growing, it is dying. This is the same message that our body receives if we do not learn and grow. We must learn and grow to age gracefully.

Ideas for communities are religious groups, education groups, schools or continuing education such as a creative writing class or professional development, business networking groups, exercise groups, country clubs, art classes, knitting groups ("stitch and bitch"), book clubs, and more. In order to find these groups, you might simply look in the local paper for events to attend or group meetings. You can look online for meet-up groups in your area. Sometimes schools or community centers offer classes in interesting topics that might interest you. Community groups or senior centers also offer exercise classes. You can even start a group easily with some friends you might already have; just pick a meeting place and a topic. The list goes on.

Moais

In Okinawa, Japan, people form *moais*. A moai is a small group of people who have known each other from a young age. They commit to each other and meet regularly for a common goal. These small groups become like a second family. The word moai means "meeting for a common purpose." Traditionally, these groups were formed for financial support. For example, if a member of a moai needed money to start a business, all members of the moai would pool their money together for the one member. However, they are not just a financial safety net. They also have a deep respect for and support each other. Currently, some Okinawans join more than one group.

The Barkada

My mother and father met each other in medical school at the University of the Philippines. They, along with their colleagues and *barkada*, meaning group of friends, came to America in the sixties. At the time, the United States needed good medical doctors and nurses as there was a shortage of them. Their barkada stayed together in their new homeland, working to build their careers and serve the medical needs here. They worked in the same hospitals, socialized together, opened offices together, went to church together, celebrated American traditions like Thanksgiving together, and attended each other's weddings and their children's weddings for the past 50 years. The common thread was their nationality, culture, vocation, and values. That barkada that they created in their student days became a support network and a new family for them halfway around the world. Many of them are thriving in their retirement. They go to the movies, go to dinner, exercise together, and have formed book clubs that meet regularly.

PURPOSE IS POWER

Having purpose in life helps you get out of bed in the morning, ready to live life with gusto. Many studies support the powerful connection between purpose and longevity. I find that patients who continue to daydream, set goals, and pursue projects and who look forward to specific tasks in their day—even something as simple as making a favorite meal or repairing an old car—are the ones who heal quicker from health setbacks.

This idea of purpose is exalted in many cultures. *Plan de vida*, translated as your "reason to live," is a Costa Rican idea focused on cultivating positivity as you age. It is not just about your vocation or how to change the world, but what you do to enjoy the world around you. What foods, activities, and actions bring you more pleasure and life energy.

A similar idea is the Japanese concept of *Ikigai*, the reason or source of why you are alive. The concept of Ikigai comes from the Heian period, which ran from 794 to 1184, in Japanese history. The Japanese word *gai* comes from the word *kai*, meaning "shell." During this time, shells were of high value. Ikigai implies that you should do what is valuable to you. You determine what is valuable to you, combining what you are good at, what you can get paid to do, what you can do to contribute to the world, and what you love to do. The ikigai is a combination of your personal mission, vocation, passion, and profession.

There is a very famous TED Talk by Simon Sinek that touches on this idea; the talk is named "Start with Why" and is about how great leaders inspire those around them to take action. The talk states that finding your why is the start or basis of fulfillment. It is what will get you up in the morning to go to work and what will have you return home at night to a safe and comforting environment.

If you do not know your purpose, and you want to live a long time, it is imperative you embark on a journey to find it. You can start with your journal and write down all the things you love to do. It could be making crafts, traveling, cooking, designing software, building bicycles, antique hunting, writing letters to the editor, following the stock market, giving massages, working out, underwater basket weaving, you name it. Do not put any limits on your list or judge yourself or that list as you write. Just write it all down.

Next, go do those things on the list. You might find that as you start to do the things on your list, you start to figure out what you love to do. You might also discover that what you once thought you were passionate about now bores you. That's okay, too; just cross it off your list. You might also find that you are multipassionate. In this modern age, many people are forging a new way of incorporating all their interests.

I know a plastic surgeon who travels every summer to different parts of the world to correct cleft palates in children. He combines his love of travel and passion for community service with his vocation. The difference he makes in the lives of children and their parents is amazing. He loves to do it and is touched by everyone he meets. He always ends his trips by touring the country he visited. He spends most of the rest of the year saving and raising money to go the following year. When you are living your life with a purpose like this, you look forward to a long life to fulfill that purpose.

My profession as a naturopathic doctor is my Ikigai. I love to connect with people, I am passionate about health. I feel in many ways, being a third-generation physician, that it is in my genes to be a doctor. I love the concept of healing and spend my life in a constant flux of working on healing for myself and others. However, fulfilling my purpose also sometimes involves some personal sacrifice and some trial and error.

For example, despite having the same amount of student loans and debts that conventional medical doctors incur, naturopathic doctors do not have a guaranteed residency or job at a hospital or clinic immediately after graduation. Like most other naturopaths, I had to start my own practice, and I learned that running a practice is the same as running a business. I didn't know the first thing about starting a business, much less running one. In order to make ends meet, I took a job as a nutritional consultant and health radio show host with a wonderful supplement company who knew I was building my practice. As I cut down one day at my job, I increased a day seeing patients.

However, once my practice started taking off, the responsibility of running a business became too stressful, and I found myself in the role of business owner more often than doctor. So I took a step back to recalibrate. I knew that it was very important to me to make sure I spend time devoted to my five daughters and at the same time I remembered how I loved to teach! Therefore, I decided to keep my practice small and manageable and fuel my other love of education by teaching at universities, other teaching institutions, and with online seminars. It has been gratifying for me to realize that more people learn about naturopathic medicine through my teaching. I have the perfect balance, and you can, too. It is just a matter of exploring, soul-searching, praying, checking in, and remaining clear on what you want and love to do.

SPIRITUAL SUPPORT

In all cultures, the idea of being connected to the sacred gives individuals an opportunity to cope with the rigor, stress, confusion, and hardships of a difficult world. People who are connected to some aspect of sacredness or spirituality will see their lives as being value-filled with an expectation that physical, emotional, and psychological pain will soon be a thing of the past. Therefore, there is a rewiring of our mental and psychological perspectives in which we see ourselves as being capable of surviving whatever challenge we may face.

Finding Social Connection Through a Spiritual Path

When people say New York City is the capital of the world, it's probably because it's a city teeming with souls from every corner of the planet. I've met people here from countries I've never heard of. My patients form a microcosm of all the thousands of faiths and spiritual communities, and I've seen that, for many, these groups are an important means of social connection. I have patients who are Catholic, pastors of a Baptist church, faithful Pentecostal congregants, Brooklynites who love the Christian mega church, practitioners of the Rastafari faith, people from the Orthodox Jewish community, and Muslims who live on the same block as their mosque. There is a woman who meditates regularly at a huge meditation center in the middle of Manhattan and one who volunteers regularly at the Bahai Center. Whatever their path, they enjoy this outlet for finding inspiration together with a like-minded group.

There are also many who do not follow a faith or a religion but have a spiritual side that is very personal to them. Often these people also find a community of like-minded souls through shared hobbies more than formal groups. But that sense of connection and mutual enthusiasm is very inspiring for them.

Whatever your spiritual outlook, there is likely a community of those who will support you and give you a framework for navigating life.

How Spirituality Can Support and Inspire

No matter your faith or religion, or absence of religion, considering your values and finding philosophical touchstones and affirmations can help you feel steady and inspired.

People with this kind of foundation are more likely to believe that everything happens for a reason and that ultimately, life itself is a teacher. So our hardships are informed by a sense that spiritual or personal growth is taking place, in good times and bad. This can be soothing, inspiring, and empowering.

Meanwhile, here are some ideas for incorporating soulful self-care, regardless of your religious leanings, throughout the day:

Try prayer: A fascinating body of research shows that prayer seems to support people regardless of whether or not the person knows they are being prayed for. Patients who are prayed for heal faster. Research is currently being conducted on the mechanisms of healing through prayer.

Set an intention: In a lot of cases, intention is everything. Set an intention for what you want to do and what you want to have, and what you want to create in your life. This is the first step to what many call "manifestation," or calling into reality what you desire.

Rest: Many cultures make time for daily downtime like siestas. Others take a weekly day of rest by observing the Sabbath. In our caffeinated American culture, it is essential to prioritize sleep and rest.

Practice love and kindness: Not just tolerate, but love and be kind to those around you. A quick conversation with the produce guy at the grocery store can actually have health benefits for both of you.

Pay it forward: Try buying coffee for strangers. Just give the barista an extra twenty dollars to pay for the next three coffees, then leave the shop. Paying kindness forward creates a ripple effect of generosity and a feeling of well-being for yourself and those you've helped.

Unplug: Power down the computer and smartphone, especially in the hours before bedtime. Read a book, dim the lights, light candles, take a bath, try a few yoga poses, or check in with your higher consciousness or higher power.

Practice gratitude: I encourage my patients to keep a gratitude journal. Writing down even two or three simple items can turn everything you have into everything you need. If you're struggling, remember the basics: "I am grateful for a bed that comforts me, a body that moves me, and the sunshine coming through the window." Gratitude can create a state of grace and calm as you recognize the good that surrounds you.

Acknowledge your successes: We forget to celebrate our successes, especially over time as our accomplishments fade into a backdrop of normalcy. The stoic philosophers noticed this thousands of years ago. How many of the realities in your life now may have been a dream to your younger self? Acknowledge your successes and enjoy a sense of accomplishment.

- Understand that relationships, socialization, and spiritual support play a significant role in longevity and quality of life.

- Relationships provide purpose, meaningful interaction, service, and connectedness.

- Most centenarians do not reach 100 in isolation.

- On the other hand, unhealthy relationships are believed to add inflammation to your body.

- Getting active in your community by volunteering, providing services, and engaging in hobbies with a group of friends all support longevity and fulfillment.

- Waking up each day with a sense of curiosity and purpose can extend your life.

- Your spirituality, whether based in formal religion or not, is very important in becoming a master ager. It provides a framework for coping with stress and can give purpose to your life.

- Engage with your family. Have dinner together, cuddle, try out the six-second kiss with your partner, become aware of how you can interact and connect with them.

- Repair, revise, reinvent, or, if you must, relinquish the toxic relationships in your life.

- Get involved in your community or tribe: Take a class, check out your local community center or senior center, or start your own club.

- Cultivate new friendships and reconnect with old ones.

- Explore your purpose and write it down.

- Cultivate a spiritual or philosophical outlook that inspires and supports you.

- Define what soulful self-care means to you and consider scheduling prayer, meditation, or other uplifting activities in your calendar.

- Greet and chat with strangers throughout your day. Consider it a form of service, self-care, or even a spiritual adventure.

1. Do you have meaningful relationships with friends and family members? Y or N (–1 points for no, 1 point for Y, 2 points for it's good, 3 points for it's great)

2. Do you eat meals with your family? Y or N (–1 point for no, 1 point for two or more times per week, 2 points for five to seven days a week)

3. Do you express affection and love regularly? Y or N (–1 point for N, 1 point for sometimes, 2 points for most times, 3 points for all the time)

4. Do any of your relationships weigh you down? Y or N (–3 points for more than three relationships, –2 points for two or more, –1 for one toxic relationship, 1 point for no toxic relationships)

5. Are you working on yourself or with a professional to heal unhealthy or challenging relationships? Y or N (–1 point for N, 1 point for Y)

6. Are you involved in a community or tribe? Y or N (–1 point for N, 1 point for every community you can think of)

7. Do you feel a sense of purpose? Y or N (–1 point for N, 1 point for Y, 2 points for actively trying to figure it out or actively reevaluating)

8. Do you consider yourself a spiritual person? Y or N (–1 point for N, 1 point for Y)

9. Do you engage in some sort of soul-enriching activity regularly (does not have to be a formal type of religion)? Y or N (–1 point for N, 1 point for Y)

10. Add a point for every quick tip or soulful self-care you engage in.

SCORE

0 points or less: I encourage you to focus on your sense of connection.

0 to 8 points: You're connected in some ways but could probably deepen your ties to community.

8 to 16 points: Impressive.

16 or above: Excellent! You're well on your way to being a super ager.

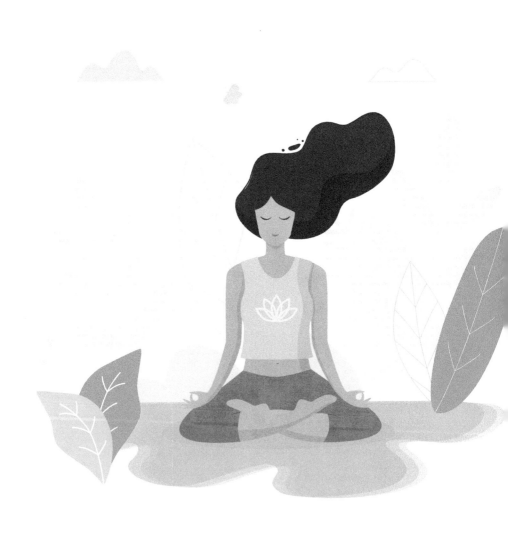

CHAPTER 5

Chill

I n a sense, our bodies have only two settings: excitement or calm. The first, the excitement setting, is also known as the "fight-or-flight" state. Our sympathetic nervous system kicks in, prepared to give us a jolt of energy to handle the dangers at hand. Conversely, when we're calm, we're operating in the para-sympathetic state, also known as the "rest-and-digest" mode.

Back in our hunting and gathering days, we would be pleasantly walking around, munching on berries, until a predator sauntered or leapt into view. To deal swiftly with our undesirable new company, our bodies produced a slew of reactive and energizing hormones—the sympathetic nervous system to the rescue.

In that fight-or-flight mode, our heart rate shoots up, our blood pressure rises, and the adrenals kick into high gear. An injection of cortisol and adrenaline—and resulting surge of energy—helped our ancestors outrun or spear the intruding carnivore. Those hormones create a surge of energy that's designed to be useful but temporary. Once the danger was resolved, we could get back to those berries.

In our modern lives, we can get stuck in sympathetic mode. Instead of the fanged predator, we have more nebulous stressors that sometimes keep our nervous and hormonal systems turned up longer than nature intended. Think of unpaid bills, pressure from a cantankerous boss, an argument with a partner, or daily traffic. You can't just throw a spear at those problems, roast them over a fire, and call it a day. I mean, you could try, but I think we can agree it wouldn't end well. So what to do instead? I'll get to that shortly.

STRESS AND THE BRAIN

Before I go into the good news about the many solutions for reducing your stress levels, it's important to understand how your brain reacts to stress. Stress, especially chronic stress, creates undesirable changes in the brain. Stress can shrink the prefrontal cortex and actually kill off brain cells. When the body undergoes stress, the amygdala receives the message and sends a signal to the hypothalamus, which is the command center in the brain that turns on the sympathetic nervous system mode I described above.

If stress is persistent and frequent, the amygdala receives messages over and over again. Just as your biceps will enlarge by lifting weights over and over, your amygdala expands due to repeated excitations. You might want bigger biceps, but you do not want a bigger amygdala. A larger, more active amygdala is conditioned to enter sympathetic mode more often and more readily.

An oversize amygdala in turn calls upon the adrenal glands, which sit on top of your kidneys, and requests more cortisol. As the hunter/gatherer parable suggests, cortisol isn't all bad. It's what wakes us up in the morning and keeps us focused on work, giving us energy throughout the earlier part of the day. It should peak at about 8 a.m. and then slowly taper off until bedtime. That's the healthy cortisol cycle. However, chronic stress leads to prolonged secretion of cortisol. This imbalanced cortisol cycle is hard on the brain and taxes the nervous system.

Furthermore, the body prioritizes survival over healing. Therefore, the mechanisms used to heal or restore the brain are put on the back burner in times of danger or perceived danger. For example, inflammation can build up in our brain, creating a sort of "tar" called amyloid plaques. Amyloid plaques need to be cleaned up if we expect to avoid Alzheimer's disease or dementia. When undergoing stress, the brain's concern is to flee from the "predator" so it will use all its energy for that purpose and leave those amyloid plaques for later.

But that's not going to be the case for you. Instead, you're on your way to becoming a plaque-free super ager, ready to chuck the stress and live a long and thriving life. Let's talk about how.

LIFESTYLE EDITS TO SLAY STRESS

Whatever qualms we might have with modernity, humans now have more opportunities to live safe, happy, lower-stress lives. Of course, there are dire situations and even life-threatening ones in modern life. However, many of us are simply stressed by everyday life.

Dealing with bills, a difficult client, or an overwhelming amount of paperwork doesn't have to push us into survival mode. Remember that many such tasks are doable, especially if you focus on problem-solving and take projects one step at a time. While your to-do list may always be there, learning to change your relationship to it is a primary task.

Enlist Your Body

Under the influence of stress or unexamined emotions, we're not likely to eat as well. We either stop eating because we lose our appetite or we grab that pastry that gives us a sugar high and the illusion that we're shifting into rest-and-digest mode. These choices made in haste can sabotage the goals of the super ager who wants to eat like a king or queen and reap all the benefits of a body flooded with nutrition.

Stop and assess: Step one is to slow down and be mindful about our food choices when stressed. This is also critical for keeping our blood sugar balanced. When our sugar drops—whether due to skipping meals or eating sweets—your adrenals kick in to create energy to keep you going. This might actually feel good at first, like a caffeine kick, but over time, your adrenal glands get tired and call upon the thyroid for help. You don't need that cycle of hormonal stress. Instead of sugar, eat healthy fats and protein. Think instead of a few nuts, handful of seeds, hummus and celery, apple and almond butter, or an avocado rolled up in a lettuce leaf with some extra-virgin olive oil and vinegar drizzled on top. These foods take longer to digest and tend to keep your blood sugar stable.

Shake it off: Next, add movement. When your system is flooded with hormones associated with the sympathetic mode, we sometimes need to burn them off the old-fashioned way, by outrunning the predator. Of course, in this case, nothing will chase you through your Zumba class. But as you move, those hormones will indeed be flushed from the body.

Add love: Another way we can change the stress response is by secreting oxytocin, the "love" hormone. There are countless ways to activate this wonderful and soothing hormone, from cuddling a pet to talking with your child to looking into your partner's eyes and thinking of all their best qualities. Write your own list and revisit it often. These loving encounters will help us enter parasympathetic mode, giving our adrenals a break and prepping our bodies for a longer, healthier, and happier life.

Practice Restorative Self-care

You see the hashtags on Facebook and Instagram: #treatyourself #loveyourself #selfcare #selfcaresunday #metime. But what does it mean to practice self-care? Here are some small and simple ways to pepper your day with calming and inspiring moments:

- Upon waking, open up the curtains and let the light in.

- Savor a tall glass of water.

- Meditate. More on that in "Meditation and Mindfulness" (page 90).

- Pray or chant to greet the day.

- Stretch or do a 10-minute walk.

- Read the transformative book *The Miracle Morning* by Hal Elrod.

Throughout the Day

- Put some essential oils into a diffuser. Citrus scents can be energizing, while rose, ylang-ylang, and cypress are perfect for calming. Do not diffuse essential oils if you have pets, as essential oils can be dangerous for animals.

- Have a 5- to 15-minute declutter session; shred old papers, put dirty clothes in the laundry bin, or find some items to add to that box for donation.

- Enjoy music you love.

- Turn on your favorite song or create a playlist of them.

- Take deep breaths.

- Call a friend.

- Take a quick walk while you catch up with that friend.

- Prepare some healthy snacks for the week.

- Make yourself smile and laugh—find a funny meme or watch a comedy show.

- Sit outside and simply observe nature or "people watch" for a few minutes.

- Make a gratitude list.

- Light a candle and dim the lights.

- Log it all in your journal.

- Write a thank-you note.

- Turn off the phone, TV, or any blue lights.

- Give yourself (or someone else) a big hug.

- Do a face mask.

- Slip into a bath.

- Read something wonderful.

- Stargaze with some herbal tea.

- Put a drop of lavender essential oil onto your pillow.

MEDITATION AND MINDFULNESS

For me, the word "meditation" used to conjure images of an old sage, preferably with a long white beard, sitting cross-legged in a temple on a mountaintop. However, in the past two decades, the practice of meditation has become mainstream, touted for its ability to promote peace, concentration, sleep, resilience, diminished anxiety, relief from depression, and a host of physical benefits such as lower blood pressure.

ABC journalist Dan Harris began practicing meditation years ago after suffering a panic attack during a live broadcast. Since then, he has written a book on the subject of meditation and how it has benefited himself and his family. He also hosts a popular weekly podcast called *10 Percent Happier* that discusses ways to meditate and researches the benefits of doing so.

There are multiple ways to meditate. It can be done in a group or alone. It can take hours or just a few minutes. It can be guided or silent. In any event, meditation can be helpful for people like you and me.

There are numerous ways to meditate. Here are a few simple suggestions to explore:

Focus meditation: First, try choosing a mantra. My favorites are: "focus," "peace," "tranquility," "power," "abundance," or "health." Or invent more interesting, unusual phrases like "rock steady" or "firelight." Use this word or phrase as your anchor; what feelings does it evoke? What thoughts do you have about it? If it's a negative thought, just acknowledge it and move on to the next thought. If you find yourself wandering away from the word, gently notice and pull yourself back to the meditation. Imagine a flame, an animal or another symbol. Or simply concentrate on your breath. See what you discover. There is no "wrong" way to mediate. Be patient with your body and mind as you begin a practice. Most of us suffer from racing thoughts or what yogis call "monkey mind." Just being still is a good place to start.

Mindfulness meditation: Close your eyes and get in a comfortable, seated position. Quietly become aware of everything happening around you. Notice the hum of traffic outside, the clock ticking, the wind through the trees, birds chirping, floors creaking, and if music is playing, notice all the instruments and notes. Use all your senses—feel the heat of the room, take note of smells and sensations. What textures are you feeling against your skin? This meditation is very grounding. It can help you relax, take in a new perspective, or conjure a feeling of balance. Try this mindfulness meditation at home, on the bus, in nature, or wherever you can find a moment for stillness.

Guided meditation: This is a beginner-friendly way to learn to meditate. There are many CDs, apps, podcasts, and downloads available today. Even Alexa and Siri have guided meditations available. These recordings use music and a soothing voice to give you meditation instructions. Most of these meditations are designed for a particular benefit such as helping you reduce stress, manifest more wealth, sleep more deeply, let go of unwanted thoughts, practice self-love, or build your confidence.

Chanting meditation: One of the most well-known chanting, or singing, meditations entails sitting comfortably and making the sound "om" on a long exhalation. Om is a universal sound that places you in tune with the cosmos. In other words, the sound tunes and balances your body, mind, and sleep. It may also help you align with your true, higher self. There may be many advantages to chanting, from the way the sound vibrations affect your nervous system to the benefits of the physical act of singing. Like mantra meditation, it's also a method of focusing the mind on a narrower range of thoughts. In this case, you're focusing on a single sound, word, or phrase. Try the "om" mantra or simply sing a phrase from a hymn, line of poetry, or spiritual text that's meaningful to you.

Spiritual meditation: Like prayer, this approach to meditation invites you to call upon the divine, as you define it. The goal is to deepen your connection to your highest source of meaning and inspiration. Take the moment to connect with your spirit by using prayer, thoughts, or the absence of thought. If you so desire, use the practice of meditation to further develop your spirituality.

What's important is not the type of meditation you do, but that you include it in your daily routine. In addition to our own well-being and health, the benefits of meditation often have a ripple effect on everyone close to us. If we're feeling calm, centered, and balanced in our energies, we can relate with more kindness toward everyone who crosses our path.

WHAT DOES HAPPINESS HAVE TO DO WITH IT?

Over the past 10 to 20 years, we've seen a rise in research into a topic that should interest all of us: happiness. What makes humans happy? It turns out that there are places in the world where people report very high levels of happiness. Citizens in these happy places experience pleasure and purpose in their daily lives.

Singapore, Denmark, and Costa Rica have been identified as three of the world's happiest places. Although seemingly very different cultures, there are common threads between them. First, all three governments place a premium on education and human development. All three boast 100 percent literacy for the children of their nations.

Second, basic needs of the people are met or attainable, which includes a priority on public health and preventive health care. Having your basic needs met, and a good foundation of education and health, means survival no longer has to be prioritized. Instead pride, pleasure, and purpose can be cultivated.

People from Singapore have a strong sense of pride knowing that if they work hard, they will get into a good school, eventually land a very good job, and attain financial security. Ambition is valued and subsequently rewarded. People feel proud of their accomplishments, and this feeling of well-being ripples out into their relationships with family and friends.

Conversely, in Denmark, the idea of ambition in order to climb a social, political, or economic ladder is frowned upon. Instead, the society focuses on equality, personal freedom, and individual expression of interests and talents. Health care and a college education are provided for all. When these basic societal needs become a right, not a privilege, people are free to pursue any career that they are passionate about. The Danish are free to find their purpose and authentic interests. As we've discussed, a sense of purpose is a major contributor to one's happiness—and longevity.

In Costa Rica, people emphasize living a slow-paced lifestyle and spending time with friends and family. They tend to be highly active in their communities with up to five or six hours a day spent socializing. They report feeling joy and pleasure. In addition, as I have mentioned, Costa Rica is also home to a large centenarian population.

I'm happy to report that an American town made the cut of one of the happiest places on earth. San Luis Obispo is a coastal town between Los Angeles and San Francisco. The town, which loves to call itself by its acronym, SLO, was designed to promote quality of life. Planners ensured that, as the town grew, it remained aesthetically pleasing with less pollution, fewer signs, wider sidewalks for walking, accessible and safe bike lanes, antismoking policies for public spaces, and more public gathering places. There are preserved green spaces that include parks, beaches, hiking trails, campsites, mountain bike trails, and wildlife preserves. The arts are supported in this town where art galleries, painting, film, orchestra, opera, and music in general are all enjoyed. People pursue their hobbies here and remind each other to take life SLO, as in "slow." There's a tremendous sense of solidarity around these values and the protection of life quality. For people of SLO, California, happiness is a top priority.

I encourage you to read more about the happiest places in the world and consider how the people there manage stress—or seem to have renounced it completely. It can be eye-opening to see how many of our tensions may be related to cultural conditioning and lifestyle habits which, with a bit of effort, we can transform for ourselves.

NATURE CONNECTIONS

We as humans are meant to live and thrive in nature. As a Brooklyn, New York, resident, I know it is more than possible to survive in this concrete jungle. However, to really get restoration, to receive real nurturing, and for optimal health, New Yorkers often need to visit and sit in one of the city's many parks, taking time to observe the trees and landscape, and/or ideally, leave the city for a day trip to the woods. It is here where we can achieve true restoration. If you live in the woods or spend a lot of time outdoors, you have an advantage.

Natural sunlight sends important messages to our brain, signaling the release of hormones in our pituitary gland and throughout our bodies in addition to producing critical hormones through our skin such as vitamin D. These cues inform our endocrine system, influencing our metabolism, stress responses, sleep cycles, and so much more. So in addition to enjoying the fresh clean air, spending time under the sky helps your body reset itself and plug back into its natural rhythms and processes. Shoot for a few hours per day or find any minutes you can—taking a call outside, instigating a walking meeting, or simply taking a tea or coffee break on a bench.

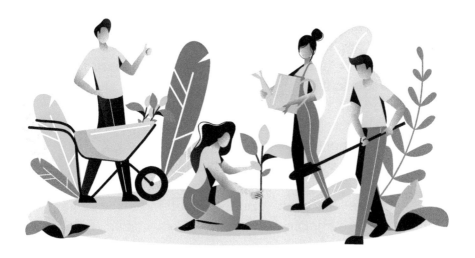

Forest Bathing

In Japan, they practice *shinrin-yoku*, meaning "taking in the forest," otherwise known as forest bathing. Forest bathing is easy to do. All we have to do is simply walk in the forest and take it all in. Notice the sights, the smells, the sounds, and all the feelings that come up. If your mind is racing with busyness, to-do lists, and stressors, gently pull your attention toward the forest and watch how the stressors disappear. Our adrenal glands and bodies will respond in turn by relaxing and letting go.

Research published in the *Journal of the American Heart Association* demonstrates that the more exposure we have to green spaces the fewer biomarkers to cardiovascular disease we will have. Time in nature is associated with lower blood pressure and reduced cardiovascular risk. Also, hospital patients, when exposed to nature, have a shortened recovery time.

As human beings, our natural habitat is nature. Taking a walk in nature can help nourish your adrenal glands by helping you slow your breath, take in clean air, move your joints, calm your thoughts, and digest stress.

Sunlight Health and Safety

An added benefit of walking through the forest is that we get to enjoy some shade. Because some of our protective ozone layer is missing, high levels of direct sun exposure can damage our skin, break down our collagen, and cause wrinkles. Too many of the sun's rays can also increase our risk for skin cancer. We want to spend a little bit of time in the sun to increase our vitamin D levels. It just has to be the right amount given your constitution and skin tone.

Research shows that 10 to 15 minutes of exposure to the sun per day minimizes the risk of sun damage and will still increase your vitamin D levels. If you expose the insides of your arms and thighs—that thin inner skin—to the sun, you will synthesize more vitamin D. In our modern lives, vitamin D deficiency is common. Therefore, supplementation of this crucial, cancer-fighting nutrient might be necessary. Your doctor can let you know whether you are deficient with a simple blood test. Sufficient vitamin D levels are equated with many health benefits.

People with high vitamin D levels have fewer colds and flus, fewer heart attacks, and decreased chances of having a stroke. Vitamin D helps facilitate more stable blood sugar levels and patients tend to be more balanced and have stronger bones, fewer hip fractures, and more protection against autoimmune disease. It may even prevent some types of cancer. For example, according to a review published in *Breast Cancer: Basic and Clinical Research*, there are over 5,000 case studies demonstrating a strong correlation between breast cancer and low vitamin D levels. Overall, we can conclude that the benefits of vitamin D supplements most definitely correlate with a longer, healthier life.

Choose to Live Restfully

In modern society, there is a de-emphasis on rest and a focus on doing. We are not human doings, we are human beings. We should give ourselves permission for a break. Consider indulging in a siesta once in a while. This gives the body more opportunity and time to heal. We are not healing when we are doing housework, running errands, or commuting to work, and certainly not when we are working. Remember, we are biological beings, not mechanical machines. We heal when we rest. To those of you who never let themselves take a nap, napping is healthy, not lazy. If you don't seem to respond well to naps, give yourself permission to go to bed early. If the body can sleep, it means the body needs sleep.

Sleep Is Your Friend

We are diurnal in nature, meaning we are awake to do most of our activities during the day and are meant to sleep at night.

A critical way to honor our natural rhythms and thereby take stress off the body is by going to sleep at the same time each night. Studies show that a bedtime at or before 10 p.m. is best. You will get deeper, more restful sleep between the hours of 10 p.m. and 6 a.m. than if you got eight hours between, say, 1 a.m. and 9 a.m. Also, it is important to note that the American Academy of Sleep Medicine (AASM) and the Sleep Research Society (SRS) developed a consensus recommendation—based on cumulative researched evidence—for the amount of sleep needed to promote optimal health in adults: seven to nine hours of sleep per night. You might need more than nine if you are a young adult or you have a sleep debt. Yes, sleep debt is a real thing, and most of us experience it at some time or other. A sleep debt refers to your body's desire to make up for lost sleep. Take note: Our deepest healing comes when we are at rest—in particular during deep sleep.

The *Journal of Sleep Research* published a summary of studies looking at people who do not get enough sleep. The study participants were required to follow strict bedtime schedules and by doing so, increased their sleep by about 20 minutes to 3 hours more of sleep. The results showed participants had decreased appetites, decreased cravings for sugar and salt, and better blood sugar maintenance. Imagine the difference you can make for your health by going to bed just 20 minutes earlier.

You will want to have a nighttime ritual to help you make the switch from parasympathetic mode to sympathetic mode. For example, brush your teeth, get in your pajamas, drink some Sleepytime tea to aid with sleep, turn the lights down low, maybe read or meditate. Just like you had a bedtime ritual as a child, you need one for yourself. You get a bonus if you recruit a family member and cuddle on the couch for a few minutes before heading to bed. You will get into parasympathetic mode quickly.

Choosing to live restfully is the opposite of choosing to live stressfully. Since stress is often a reaction, it will take the action steps outlined in the previous paragraph to help you manage stress or at least interrupt it to live a longer better quality of life.

- Remember, as humans we are in one of two modes: the parasympathetic mode (rest and digest) or the sympathetic mode (fight or flight).

- The goal is to moderate stress by avoiding getting stuck in sympathetic mode.

- You can diminish stress by practicing restorative self-care and eating the right foods.

- Meditation is a huge tool for managing stress.

- Meditation does not have to be complicated, and there are many ways to meditate.

- Nature is very important for helping you manage stress and remain healthy. Exposure to nature is important, and consciously placing yourself in nature and working in concert with your natural circadian rhythms is very important to nurture your adrenal glands and control stress.

- Happiness is also an important factor that is associated with managing stress.

- Try out all or any of the self-care practices outlined in this chapter.

- Try meditating, starting with one minute. Check out meditation apps for help.

- Prioritize sleep. Aim to be in bed by 10 p.m.

- Connect with nature. Schedule a nature walk or forest bath. Take care of some houseplants or office plants. Plants are especially important if you live in the city.

- Have protein at your meals to balance your blood sugar and prevent stress from blood sugar highs or lows.

1. Do you easily feel edgy or anxious? Y or N (−2 points for Y and 1 point for N)

2. Are you able to bounce back from tense or anxiety-provoking experiences quickly? Y or N (2 points for Y and −2 points for N)

3. Give yourself 1 point for every self-care tip you employed this week.

4. Did you meditate this week? Y or N (3 points for three or more times, 2 points for two or more times, 1 point for one time)

5. Did you get 7 to 9 hours of sleep each night of this week? Y or N (4 points for seven times this week, 3 points for five or more times this week, 2 points for four or more times, 1 point for three or more times, -2 for two or less times)

6. Did you spend some time in nature this week? Y or N (3 points for three or more times, 2 points for two or more times, 1 point for one time)

7. Are you supplementing with vitamin D3? Y or N (1 point for Y, −1 point for N)

8. Are you having protein with meals and snacks? Y or N (1 point for Y and −1 point for N)

SCORE

Below 0 points: It's time to consider your stress management strategy.

0 to 8 points: That's a start, but you need to find more time for self-care and relaxation.

8 to 16 points: You're pretty chill. Keep it up.

16 or above: Hey, stress master! Please teach others.

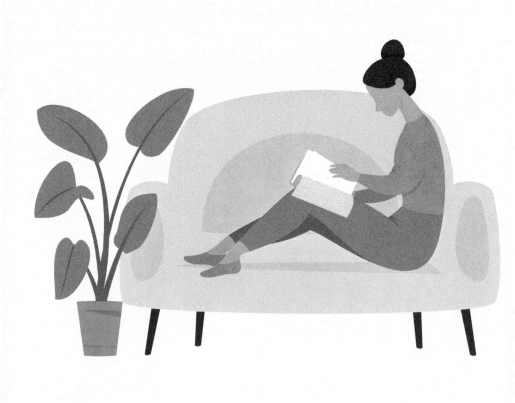

CHAPTER 6

Super-Aging Action Plan

Welcome to your personal super-aging action plan. In this chapter we will go step by step to help you define your goals. Here we will create new habits for you to become a super ager. It is important to create habits that you can implement in your daily life. Without implementation, then everything you learned in this book becomes simply information. But information is not transformation. The real transformation can begin now. You will be adding more life into your years, body, and brain.

SET AN INTENTION

Setting an intention is like planting a seed. Without that first step, it's hard for us to direct our energies. So let's create your intention so you can clarify your goals and plan.

Self-inquiry will help you set an intention for the coming months and years of your life. To begin this introspection, please find or purchase a health journal. There are certainly many app options available. Or if you prefer to write the old-fashioned way, a paperbound journal can be a treasured diary as well. You could find a beautiful journal and spend some money on it. For some of us, investing in something means we're more likely to use it. There are gorgeous leather-bound journals—or others with handmade or high-quality thick paper. You could find one with inspirational quotes or a meaningful picture on the front. However, if a fancy journal is intimidating, if it makes you fear writing in it, consider taking a simpler route. Pick up a cheap spiral-bound or composition notebook at the drugstore.

In this journal, we will design the plan. Think of your health journal as a fruition system—a tool for helping ideas become actions. It will help you keep your health goals alive and anchored to reality versus swimming around in your head. Our health journal helps us see ourselves accurately, keep track of our habits, and stay accountable and inspired whenever we hit a bump or fall back into unhelpful habits.

Because I am a naturopath, many of my patients are surprised to hear that I also sometimes find it challenging to stay healthy and keep up my best habits. To be honest, it is not that easy for me. Keeping a journal helps. My health journal is now an integral part of my own self-care program, and I look forward to revisiting it. The journal helps me see my efforts, acknowledge my progress along the way, and correct my course swiftly when I need to.

At this point in the book, you may be thinking about your life and whether you live the life of a super ager. You may be asking if you have what it takes to age as gracefully, energetically, and powerfully as you'd like? Remember, this journey is about progress, not perfection. Contemplate whether you feel you're ready to age brilliantly, with a spring in your step, veggies in the fridge, and a deep love of life. Or will you slide back into unconscious habits, perhaps getting carried along by the culture around you, whether healthy or not? Or are you willing to bring your conscious awareness to all facets of your life and choose to do your best to live well?

Where would you like your life to take you in the next three years? How do you see yourself? How would you like your new healthier life to look now that you've learned more about the possibility of living not just a long life, but a robust life with a strong body and mind? What you get out of the next three years of your life will determine the three after that, and so on. Before you know it, you're 100 years old and still cutting a rug at that tango class.

Consider what inspires you to live your definition of a robust and vibrant life. Think about your source of purpose, your daydreams, the experiences you long to have in the near and not-so-near future. This vision will become the fuel that activates and sustains your health journey. Your why has to be strong enough to pull you forward into healthier habits. My why is that I want to create and enjoy amazing experiences with my children and their children.

It is important to set goals and dreams for the current stage of your life, at every single age. A study conducted by Dr. Gail Matthews, a professor at Dominican University of California, demonstrated that you are 42 percent more likely to achieve a goal if you write it down. Before you set goals, dream a little. Put something down on paper.

Pull out your health journal, reflect, and write down the answers to these questions. If you find it hard to answer them, don't be discouraged. This may actually be the trickiest self-assessment in the book for some. Also recognize that your answers may change over time, so I encourage you to revisit these questions often, invoking fresh intentions, inspirations, and new understanding of yourself and your wishes for this precious life:

Self-Assessment Questions:

- What really matters to me?
- Who matters to me? Who do I spend my time with and why?
- What would I like to be doing more of?
- What do I feel passionate about—or look forward to on a regular basis?
- What is my why—my source of purpose?
- Where would I most like to live?
- What hobbies and fun things do I enjoy?
- What do I like to do for rest and relaxation?
- What are some new lifestyle habits I could consider adopting?
- How would I like to feel?
- What will my life look like in 3 years?
- What will my life look like in 10 years?
- What will I be like at age 100?

INVITE YOUR TRIBE

As you know by now, research consistently points out the role of culture, community, and social groups and how they influence our health. Your health is better when you are part of a community. It is the idea that all boats rise (or sink) together.

It can be a good idea to enlist your friends and family in your health goals. You do not exist in a vacuum. Conversation with your friends and family and the way you spend time together helps establish a new part of your collective health culture. With conversation, you enroll them in your mission—and invite them to join you. Friends and family now become your resources. Resources take on many forms; maybe they will become an encourager, a coach, a facilitator, or perhaps they will decide to join you. Perhaps they want to add more life to their years, their body, and their brain. Now that you exist as a super-ager team, you can support and inspire each other. There are many ways to bring friends, family, neighbors, and others in your community on board with you. Start simple:

- Start a walking group.

- Join a book club.

- Initiate a weekly friends' tea for social connection.

- Create a knit-and-sip group.

- Start a hobby and join online groups around the community (quilting community, restoring furniture community, planner community, car and automobile community, etc.).

- Create a Super Agers Club.

Be powerful in this journey. It is a generous act to share with those around you about what you are up to. You might have to step out of your comfort zone and be vulnerable. Being powerful means allowing others to contribute as well. Accept their resources. Networking is a powerful action toward accomplishing your goals.

WRITE YOUR PLAN

Your health journal now becomes a creative tool. Feel free to give it a fun name. Perhaps it's your Super Ager Journal or Magic Maker Notebook or Healing and Enlightenment Journal—whatever suits your personality and personal mission. Whatever you choose to call it, use it to record your vision, fill in answers to your self-assessment questions, write out milestones, and keep track of how you're feeling. Your journal becomes a tool by which you keep your goals alive in reality.

First, go ahead and review the self-assessment questions you answered in your journal in the earlier section. We are going to rewrite the answers to questions so that they are in the form of goals.

- What really matters to you?
- Who matters to you? Who is around you?
- What would you like to be doing?
- What do you feel passionate about?
- What is your why?
- Where will you live?
- What hobbies and fun things do you enjoy?
- What do you like to do for rest and relaxation?
- What are some new lifestyle habits you might consider doing?
- How would you like to feel?
- What will your life look like in 3 years?
- What will your life look like in 10 years?
- What will you be like at age 100?

Next, think about the four areas covered in this book:

- Movement
- Eat Real Food
- Connect
- Chill

Also, ask yourself, what else is important to me?

This category is for you to make your own. Use it to write any goals related to your purpose, personal mission, dreams, unfinished business, or more specific health goals.

How to Set Goals That Stick

Research finds that the best goals—the ones most likely to produce results—are doable, actionable, measurable, and easy to track. Consider setting some S.M.A.R.T. goals. Here's what that means:

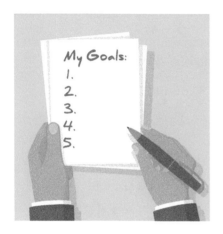

S is for Specific: Don't say, "I want to drink more water," say the specific amount. You need to drink half your weight in ounces, so if you weigh 150 pounds. Write down, "I will drink 75 ounces of water per day."

M is for Measurable: To simply state, "I want to lose some weight," doesn't give enough information. Try to get the numbers down. For example, "I want to lose 26 pounds in six months." This is much more measurable and creates a jumping-off point. From here, you can break down the goal even further into smaller daily and/or weekly increments.

A is for Achievable: Everyone starts at their own pace—meet your body where it is. For folks who do not currently exercise, just getting to the gym or creating a walking plan might be a solid first step. Others may want to level up their tennis game. Some may want to lift more weights or run a few more miles. As long as your sights are set on your own progress, you will gain a sense of accomplishment. Celebrate the little victories that keep you going.

R is for Relevant: Your methods should mirror your goal. If you've made the goal of sleeping and relaxing more, then joining another committee or signing up for an active hobby like race-car driving—while perhaps rewarding—could undermine your goal.

T is for Time: Give yourself a date and schedule it in the calendar.

Here are a few examples of S.M.A.R.T. goals:

- I will drink 75 ounces of water every day this month.
- I will be able to do three sets of bicep curls using 10-pound weights, comfortably, three months from now.
- I will take two 10-minute walks during the workday.
- I will eat green vegetables daily, have beans three times per week, exercise for 25 minutes five days per week, and have all these habits in place by May 1st.

Now you have a plan and are a force to be reckoned with. Simply by writing down your authentic goals, you are halfway to achieving your aim.

SHIELDS UP: AVOIDING
ENVIRONMENTAL TOXINS

Never in the history of the world has the human race ever had to deal with the amount of toxic chemicals we are dealing with today. There are more and more chemicals created and introduced into our environment every year. Industries in the United States reported in 1998 that 6.5 trillion tons of 9,000 different chemicals were man-ufactured—and trillions of tons of chemicals are dumped yearly. Can you imagine how many more chemicals have been introduced since then?

While our bodies are adaptable and built for daily detoxification, we should help them by lowering our exposure. The following is a list of environmental toxins and what we can do to avoid them.

ELECTROMAGNETIC FREQUENCIES (EMFS)

Electromagnetic frequencies (EMFs) or radiation from cell phone use is fairly new. I remember being in medical school in the year 2000, looking down into the courtyard from my dorm room window, seeing a doctor on a cell phone, and thinking, "What happened to his beeper?" There is some evidence that cell phone usage is safe and does not promote cancer or tumors. However, radio fre-quency radiation toxicity, such as from the sound and the radiation from cell phones, recently has been declared carcinogenic by the WHO International Agency for Research on Cancer.

It appears that the longer the exposure, the worse the damage, as even five minutes with the cell phone close to your ear could alter blood-brain permeability. The jury is still out, however, on the safety of texting and use of hands-free equipment. Consider unplugging as often as you can, but definitely consider unplugging a couple hours before bedtime. Also, be sure to place your phone across the room, or in another room altogether, when you sleep. As much as you can, speak on the phone when it is on speaker, in front of you, rather than holding it up to your ear.

HAND SANITIZER AND ANTIBACTERIAL SOAPS

Hand sanitizer and antibacterial soaps are another newly introduced vehicle for chemical contaminants. I have five daughters, and when my third daughter entered school, hand sanitizer was on the list of school supplies to bring to the teachers. This was a new concept, as it had never been on the list prior to that year. It seemed to be flying off the shelves in the dollar and office supply stores. Antibacterial hand sanitizer and soap will kill not only the bad bacteria on your skin, but the good bacteria as well. Killing your good bacteria essentially leaves you devoid of immunity.

Furthermore, using hand sanitizer encourages bacterial resistance, rendering us defenseless to evolved bad bacteria. These antibacterial soaps also contain triclosan, which appears to be toxic to living cells and toxic to our genes, causing cell mutations that may affect our children and grandchildren. Readily absorbed through the skin and into the bloodstream, triclosan is also a hormone disruptor, affecting reproductive hormone activity and the ability to metabolize thyroid hormones.

In 2016, the FDA banned the use of triclosan in over-the-counter sanitizers and washes. Triclosan has been found in our rivers and lakes, human breast milk, and urine. Use regular, old-fashioned soap instead of hand sanitizer. Do not pick antibacterial hand soap or dish soap.

Phthalates have been dubbed "obesogens" by the scientific community because, as the nickname suggests, phthalates contribute to obesity. Phthalates are solvents used in cosmetic fragrances in order to extend the aromatic strength. They appear to contribute to obesity by increasing metabolic set points, masking satiety, and regulating appetite. While phthalates are in fragrances and perfume oils, they are not in essential oils. Stop using dryer sheets. Look for unscented creams, lotions, conditioner, and shampoo. If you like delicious smells, but don't like dangerous chemicals, put a couple of drops of essential oils in your unscented toiletries or your laundry soap.

Xenoestrogens, or false estrogens, have really started to affect us in the last two decades. These are compounds that mimic some of the activity of estrogens in the human body.

Estrogens, considered the "female" hormones, are responsible for developing women's breasts and thighs, fertility, and reproduction. They also control moods and protect our bones. However, false forms in excess can promote certain health problems. The incidence of infertility and fibroids in women is on the rise. According to the National Institutes of Health, the number of adolescent boys with gynecomastia—male breasts—is now up to 50 percent.

These false estrogens are pervasive. They are in facial creams and cosmetics to plump up the face. They are in our plastics. When my first daughter was a baby, my husband and I brought home what we thought was the best baby bottle. When my second daughter was born, we went to the baby store and saw that the packaging on the same brand of baby bottles said, "Now BPA-free!" BPA or bisphenol A contains xenoestrogens and is found in soft plastics like plastic wrap, food storage containers, water bottles, shower curtains, and the lining of canned foods.

The good news is that, with a little effort, you can avoid it. Use glass food containers or porcelain to store your leftovers. Stainless steel and glass water bottles are readily available. Get cloth shower curtains to replace the plastic ones. And, as some of our elder Blue Zone inhabitants do, soak your dried beans and cook them versus using canned beans. Speaking of food, estrogen is fed to chickens to speed their growth to adulthood. It gives them bigger breasts and thighs. Cows are given hormones to make more milk at a rate that can fill up hundreds of gallon jugs for the market rather than the one calf they are lactating for.

Xenoestrogenic pesticides sprayed on vegetables emit hormonal signals that trick pests into thinking other pests are present and mating, so they should stay away. One more reason to eat organic.

WATER CONTAMINANTS

Our tap water is contaminated. For example, New York City tap water has been deemed some of the best quality tap water in the world. And, it might be, when it comes out of the water-processing plant. However, next it has to run through at least a couple of miles of pipes that run through the city and through your building. Most pipes in NYC buildings are not maintained.

Therefore, by the time it exits the faucet, it is contaminated with microplastics, sediment, and heavy metals, including lead. In 2009, a report came out that there were traces of painkillers and DEET, an insect repellent, in the tap water. In 2013, a report came out that there were 14 different types of drugs—mostly antidepressants—detected in New York City tap water. So if you are on the fence about drinking tap water, or you are confused about which reports to believe, why not just filter your water? There are some amazing water filters out there, but even the cheapest carbon filter will help.

DIOXINS

Dioxins are produced with chlorine in waste sanitation. It is what whitens things like paper, napkins, paper towels, toilet paper, and diapers. By the time a baby reaches a year old, most have exceeded the U.S. and European standards for safe dosage. Consider supporting paper companies that make dioxin-free diapers. While these more natural diapers aren't snowy white in color, your baby looks cute no matter the diaper on their little tush.

CLEANING CHEMICALS

Cleaning chemicals can actually make your house dirtier. Conventional chemical cleaners might take away dirt or grime, but they leave the surfaces in your home covered with a layer of chemicals that can contain many known toxins. Indoor air pollution is on the rise, and cleaning products can also contribute to it.

There are plenty of safer, simpler cleaning products on the market today. There is also good old-fashioned vinegar, baking soda, and water to use as cleaning agents. For a healthier home, you might consider switching over to these basic alternatives.

Other simple things you can do to support a cleaner indoor environment is pull up wall-to-wall carpeting. Carpets harbor more than forty chemicals left over from their production. Once the chemicals off-gas, carpets become a haven for dust and dirt. Another way you can keep your house cleaner is leave your shoes at the door and run around in your bare feet or put on indoor slippers. If shoes off at the door seems unrealistic, then at least have a no-shoes-in-the-bedroom rule. Then you know that for at least eight hours a day, you are not breathing in pollutants from your shoes.

PCBS (POLYCHLORINATED BIPHENYLS)

PCBs (polychlorinated biphenyls) are chemicals that were used in refrigerators and electrical equipment. Although they were banned in the United States in 1979, we still find PCBs in rivers, fish, human fat tissue, and breast milk. I am not saying avoid breastfeeding. However, simply be aware. Read labels, of course. Consider undergoing a safe detox one to four times a year, especially before getting pregnant or before breastfeeding. Do not undergo a detox while pregnant or breastfeeding.

Please look in the resources section at the end of the book for more support in living a toxin-free life (page 122).

REPEAT, REVISE & RENEW AT ANY AGE

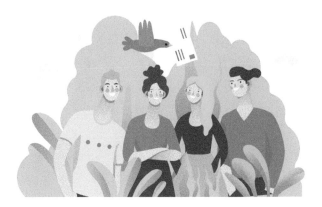

Aging brilliantly is a long-term project, and I hope it's one that inspires, uplifts, and fulfills you. After all, aging well is a source of pride, purpose, and passion in itself. So I invite you to stay in action. Information alone is not transformation. Transformation happens when you let the information inspire you. Then set an intention. Then take action. Only then will you experience the miracle of transformation.

As you take action, you will need to track your progress. See below for a list of items to track in your Super Agers Journal. Keeping a health journal teaches you to become more aware of yourself and helps you identify patterns and changes in your well-being.

Eat like a super ager: Be aware of the food and drinks you choose each day by keeping a diet diary. Write down everything that passes through your mouth. You might be surprised by what you discover. You can't make changes until you know what you're choosing now.

Make friends with water—all day: How many ounces do you need to drink? Draw pictures of a line of 8-ounce glasses.

Check off a glass every time you drink one. There is a fun app called Plant Nanny that will help keep you on track by watching if your "plant" is growing or wilting according to the amount of water you drink.

Study yourself: Headache, fatigue, constipation, diarrhea, etc. Writing them down can help you identify lifestyle habits associated with these symptoms. Look for patterns in when and how these symptoms appear. If they persist, talk to a doctor or nutritionist about what could be the issue.

Get in touch with your emotions: Feeling irritable, weepy, joyful? It's important to pay attention. One of my patients had no idea that his poor health was contributing to his horrible moods until he started eating better and taking better care of himself. He can still be sarcastic, but now fully admits how jolly he has become since working on his physical health.

Observe your nightly dreams and your daydreams: Writing down nightly dreams improves your memory and can bring insight into the subconscious. You may want to write them down first thing in the morning when they are still fresh in your mind. Also write down the daydreams and hopes you have while awake. What is the vision or dream you are holding for yourself? It's healthy to use your imagination.

Weather and mood tracking: Many people find that their moods, energy levels, or powers of concentration fluctuate with the seasons or the weather. This can give you significant information and insight into your health. If you feel depressed in winter months, for example, track your moods and consider discussing it with your doctor if you have concerns.

Steps or miles: Track your steps, miles, or workouts. Record how you feel after a hike or a dance class to learn the type of movement that's making you joyful and energized.

I encourage you to reexamine and revisit your health journal to update and reset your goals. Review and make sure your
why is still relevant. You might find that you accomplished your
goals earlier than you thought and you need to set new ones.
On the other hand, you might find that your goals were too lofty,
and you may choose to take it down a notch, so that your goal is
more attainable. Remember that living well is a journey, not
a destination. There will be trial and error.

This path is a chance for learning, self-knowledge, and
growth. It is natural for us to be in a constant state of growth.
No matter what your age, it's never too late to begin. Learning
is lifelong, and people can change their life or habits at any
moment. I'd like to close this book with some final inspiring
stories of people who have accomplished—or regained—excellent health in the second half of their lives.

Tao Porchon-Lynch is 101 years old and is the oldest living
yoga teacher. She didn't start teaching until she was 49 years
old. Prior to this career change, she had been an actress, televi-
sion producer, competitive ballroom dancer, and respected wine
connoisseur. She is a published author whose books have won
international awards. In 2015, she appeared on Season 10 of
America's Got Talent. Tao Porchon-Lynch has been quoted as
saying, "I will practice yoga until my last breath."

Stamatis Moraitis was a Greek veteran who came to the
United States in 1943. He lived in Port Jefferson, New York, for
a time and later moved to Florida with his Greek American wife
and had three children. One day, in 1976, he became short
of breath. From his recollection, nine doctors confirmed the
diagnosis of lung cancer and advised that his time was short.
Stamatis was in his 60s at the time, and his children were
adults. He and his wife moved back to Ikaria so he could live
out his final days in his hometown. They moved into his childhood home with his elderly parents.

At first, he stayed in bed, weak and exhausted, awaiting the
end. However, he started feeling better. So he began attending
services at the local church. Then, his childhood friends caught

wind that he had moved back and started showing up at his house with bottles of wine. "Might as well die happy," Stamatis thought. But he didn't die. He ended up planting and tending a vegetable garden and then adding rooms onto his parents' home. He lived there until he eventually died in 2013. He may have been 98 or 102; Stamatis could not recall his birth date.

Ernestine Shepherd is an 81-year-old female bodybuilder. She was motivated by her twin sister to start bodybuilding at age 56. In 2010, she first set the record for Oldest Female Body Builder in the *Guinness Book of World Records*. She set the record again in 2016.

AND ON YOU GO

Congratulations on your commitment to living a long, healthy, vibrant life on your terms. Make sure to celebrate your commitment and future accomplishments. Acknowledge them by writing in your journal.

May you inspire those around you. We set examples for each other and our healthy choices contribute to and support the health culture and our human community.

As you set intentions, practice over and over again, and attain new goals, you will create more and more habits that will come to you naturally as a super ager. Your practice will propel you until you are a master of aging, putting more life in your years, your body, and your brain.

May you be blessed on your health journey. You are now armed with multiple tools for protecting your vitality and living the life of your dreams for years to come. You know what to do!

GLOSSARY

Barkada: Filipino slang term for "gang of youth," "lazy to study," or "our group/our squad"

Blue Zones: regions of the world where Dan Buettner claims people live much longer than average. The five Blue Zone areas are Okinawa, Japan; Sardinia, Italy; Ikaria, Greece; Nicoya Peninsula, Costa Rica; and Loma Linda, California.

Dynapenia: loss of power due to age-related muscle loss

Epigenetics: the study of heritable changes in gene function that do not involve changes in DNA sequence

Hara hachi bu: Japanese saying meaning "belly eight parts full" or a practice of eating until you are 80 percent full

Ikigai: Japanese word meaning "The valuable source of why you are alive" or your life's purpose

Lola: Filipino "Grandma" or the Tagalog word for grandmother

Microbiome: a community of microorganisms, such as bacteria, fungi, and viruses, that inhabit a particular environment and especially the collection of microorganisms living in or on the human body

Moai: Japanese term meaning "meeting for a common purpose" or lifelong friends

Plan de vida: Costa Rican saying that stands for "why I wake up in the morning" or a soul's purpose or plan

Sarcopenia: reduction in skeletal muscle mass due to aging

Shinrin-yoku: Japanese phrase for "taking in the forest" or forest bathing

Vis medicatrix naturae: Latin phrase "The healing power of nature" or the innate natural ability of the body to heal itself

RESOURCES

The Blue Zones:
Go to Bluezones.com.

Naturopathic Medicine:
Go to Naturopathic.org.

Practitioners:
To find a naturopathic doctor such as Dr. Selassie in your area, go to Naturopathic.org and click "Find a Doctor" on the overhead tab.

For a functional medicine doctor, go to FunctionalMedicine.org and enter your location to find a practitioner near you.

Education:
Go to Aanmc.org to learn about naturopathic medical schools.

Go to Natmedcoach.com for webinars for practitioners and patients.

Go to Schoolafm.com if you are a practitioner and want to learn more about Functional Medicine.

Detoxification:
Want to learn more about toxins and how to get rid of them?

Read *Clean, Green, and Lean: Get Rid of the Toxins that Make You Fat*
by Dr. Walter Crinnio

Read *Clean Skin from Within: The Spa Doctor's Two-Week Program to Glowing, Naturally Youthful Skin*
by Dr. Trevor Cates

Want to undergo a safe online program for detoxification?
Go to Doctorselassie.com/devotional-detox-program.

REFERENCES

Andrade, Chittaranian, and Rajiv Radhakrishnan. "Prayer and Healing: A Medical and Scientific Perspective on Randomized Controlled Trials." *Indian Journal of Psychiatry* 51 (October–December 2009): 247–253, doi: 10.4103/0019-5545.58288.

Astin, John A., Elaine Harkness, and Edzard Ernst. "The Efficacy of 'Distant Healing': A Systematic Review of Randomized Trials." *Annals of Internal Medicine* 132 (2000): 903–10. doi:10.732 6/0003-4819-132-11-200006060-00009.

Atoum, Manar, and Foad Alzoughool. "Vitamin D and Breast Cancer: Latest Evidence and Future Steps." Breast Cancer: *Basic and Clinical Research* (December 2017): 11 published online. doi:10.1177/1178223417749816.

Baan, Robert, Yan Grosse, Beatrice Lauby-Secretan, Fatiha El Ghissassi, Veroniquw Bouvard, Lamia Benbrahim-Tallaa, Neela Guha, et al. "Carcinogenicity of Radiofrequency Electromagnetic Fields." *The Lancet Oncology* 12, no. 7 (July 2011): 624–626 doi: https://doi.org/10.1016/S1470-2045(11)70147-4.

Bedoux, Gilles, Benoit Roig, Olivier Thomas, Virginie Dupont, Barbara Le Bot. "Occurrence and Toxicity of Antimicrobial Tri-closan and By-Products in the Environment." *Environmental Science and Pollution Research* 19, no. 4 (May 2012): 1044–65. doi: 10.1007/s11356-011-0632-z.

Broadney, Miranda M., Britni R. Belcher, David A. Berrigan, Robert J. Brychta, Ira L. Tigner Jr., Faizah Shareef, Alexia Papachristopoulou, et al. "Effects of Interrupting Sedentary Behavior with Short Bouts of Moderate Physical Activity on Glucose Tolerance in Children with Overweight and Obesity: A Randomized Crossover Trial." *Diabetes Care* 41, no. 10 (October 2018): 2220–2228. doi: 10.2337/dc18-0774.

Buettner, Dan, and Sam Skemp. "Blue Zones: Lessons from the World's Longest Lived." *American Journal of Lifestyle Medicine* 10, no. 5 (2016): 318–321. doi: 10.1177/1559827616637066.

Buettner, Dan. "The Secrets of Long Life." *National Geographic Magazine.* November 2005, 2–27.

Buettner, Dan. *The Blue Zones: Lessons for Living Longer from the People Who've Lived the Longest.* New York: National Geographic Books, 2008.

Buettner, Dan. *Thrive: Finding Happiness the Blue Zones Way.* New York: National Geographic Books, 2010.

Carnegie Mellon University. "Stress Contributes to Range of Chronic Diseases, Review Shows." *ScienceDaily.* ScienceDaily, October 10, 2007. https://www.sciencedaily.com/ releases/2007/10/071009164122.htm.

Elrod, Hal. *The Miracle Morning: The Not-So-Obvious Secret Guaranteed to Transform Your Life (Before 8am).* N.p.: Hal Elrod International, Inc., 2012.

Federation of American Societies for Experimental Biology (FASEB). "Families That Eat Together May Be the Healthiest, New Evidence Confirms." *ScienceDaily.* April 23 2012. https:// www.sciencedaily.com/releases/2012/04/120423184157.htm.

Gardner, Sarah, and Dave Albee. "Study Focuses on Strategies for Achieving Goals, Resolutions." (2015). News. 266. https:// scholar.dominican.edu/news-releases/266.

Godman, Heidi. "Adopt a Mediterranean Diet Now for Better Health Later." *Harvard Health Blog.* November 6, 2013. https://www.health.harvard.edu/blog/adopt-a-mediterranean -diet-now-for-better-health-later-201311066846.

Gomes, Bruno A. Q., João P. B. Silva, Camila F. R. Romeiro, Sávio M. Dos Santos, Caroline A. Rodrigues, Pricila R.

Gonçalves, Joni T. Sakai, et al. "Neuroprotective Mechanisms of Resveratrol in Alzheimer's Disease: Role of SIRT1." *Oxidative Medicine and Cellular Longevity.* 30 (2018): 2018. doi: 10.1155/2018/8152373.

Govindaraju Diddahally, Gil Atzmon, and Nir Barzilai. "Genetics, Lifestyle and Longevity: Lessons from Centenarians." *Applied and Translational Genomics* 4, no. 4 (2015): 23–32. doi: 10.1016/j.atg.2015.01.001.

Guo, Yue-liang L., Mei-Lin L. Yu, Chen-Chin Hsu, and Walter J. Rogan. "Chloracne, Goiter, Arthritis, and Anemia after Polychlorinated Biphenyl Poisoning: 14-Year Follow-Up of the Taiwan Yucheng Cohort." *Environmental Health Perspectives* 107, no. 9 (1999): 715–719. doi:10.1289/ehp.99107715.

Hair, Marilyn, and Jon Sharpe. "Fast Facts about the Human Microbiome." The Center for Ecogenetics and Environmental Health, University of Washington. http://depts.washington.edu/ceeh/downloads/FF_Microbiome.pdf.

Harris, Dan. *10% Happier: How I Tamed the Voice in My Head, Reduced Stress Without Losing My Edge, and Found Self-Help That Actually Works—A True Story.* New York: Dey Street Books, 2014.

Harvard Women's Health Watch. "Putting Off Retirement May Benefit Your Brain, Health, and Longevity." Harvard Health Publishing, Harvard Medical School. September 2017. https://www.health.harvard.edu/staying-healthy/putting-off-retirement-may-benefit-your-brain-health-and-longevity.

Hedin, Charlotte R., Christopher J. van der Gast, Andrew J. Stagg, James O. Lindsay, and Kevin Whelan. "The Gut Microbiota of Siblings Offers Insights into Microbial Pathogenesis of Inflammatory Bowel Disease." *Gut Microbes* 8, no. 4 (2017): 359–365. doi: 10.1080/19490976.2017.1284733.

Henst, Rob H. P., Paula R. Pienaar, Laura C. Roden, Dale E. Rae. "The Effects of Sleep Extension on Cardiometabolic Risk Factors: A Systematic Review." *Journal of Sleep Research* 28, no. 6 (2019) doi: 10.1111/jsr.12865.

Herskind, Anne Matthew, M. McGue, Niels V. Holm, Thorkild I. Sørensen, Bent Harvald, and James W. Vaupel. "The Heritability of Human Longevity: A Population-Based Study of 2,872 Danish Twin Pairs Born 1870–1900." *Human Genetics* 97, no. 3 (March 1996): 319-323. doi:10.1007/bf02185763.

Hill, Jacob, and Wendy Hodsdon. "In Utero Exposure and Breast Cancer Development: An Epigenetic Perspective." *Journal of Environmental Pathology,Toxicology and Oncology* 33, no. 3 (2014): 239–245. Doi: 10.1615/ JEnvironPatholToxicolOncol.2014011005.

Hollenberg, Norman K., Naomi D. Fisher, and Marjorie L. McCullough. "Flavanols, the Kuna, Cocoa Consumption, and Nitric Oxide." *Journal of the American Society of Hypertension* 3, no. 2 (2009): 105–12. doi: 10.1016/j.jash.2008.11.001.

Holt-Lunstad, Julianne, Timothy B. Smith, and J. Bradley Layton. "Social Relationships and Mortality Risk: A Meta-Analytic Review." *PLOS Medicine* 7, no. 7 (July 2010): e1000316. doi: 10.1371/journal.pmed.1000316.

Jefferis, Barbara J., Tessa J. Parsons, Claudio Sartini, et al. "Objectively Measured Physical Activity, Sedentary Behaviour and All-Cause Mortality in Older Men: Does Volume of Activity Matter More Than Pattern of Accumulation?" *British Journal of Sports Medicine* 53, no.16 (2019): 1013–1020. doi: 10.1136/ bjsports-2017-098733.

Klatz, Ronald, MD, DO, and Robert Goldman, MD, PHD, DO, FAASP. "Anti-Aging Medicine: There can be no Anti-Aging without Detoxification." *Townsend Letter*. April 2016. https:// www.townsendletter.com/April2016/antiage0416.html.

Laursen, Martin F., Gitte Zachariassen, Martin I. Bahl, Anders Bergström, Arne Høst, Kim F. Michaelsen, and Tine R. Licht. "Having Older Siblings Is Associated with Gut Microbiota Development During Early Childhood." *BMC Microbiology* 15 (2015): 154. doi: 10.1186/s12866-015-0477-6.

Mariotti, Agnese. "The Effects of Chronic Stress on Health: New Insights into the Molecular Mechanisms of Brain-Body Communication." *Future Science* OA 1, no.3 (2015): 3. doi: 10.4155/fso.15.21.

Negrete-Corona, J., J. C. Alvarado Soriano, and L. A. Reyes Santiago. "Hip fracture as risk factor for mortality in patients over 65 years of age. Case-control study." *Acta Ortopedica Mexicana* 28, no. 6 (2014): 352–362. https://www.ncbi.nlm.nih.gov /pubmed/26016287.

Passwater, Richard *A. Live Better, Longer: The Science Behind the Amazing Health Benefits of OPC.* Laguna Beach, CA: Basic Health Publications, Inc., 2007.

Paterni, Ilaria, Carlotta Granchi, and Filippo Minutolo. "Risks and Benefits Related to Alimentary Exposure to Xenoestrogens." Critical *Reviews in Food Science and Nutrition* 57, no.16 (2017): 3384–3404. doi: 10.1080/10408398.2015.1126547.

Peper, Martin, Martin Klett, and Rudolf Morgenstern. "Neuropsychological Effects of Chronic Low-Dose Exposure to Polychlorinated Biphenyls (PCBs): A Cross-Sectional Study." *Environmental Health* 4 (2005): 22. doi: 10.1186/1476-069X-4-22.

Qin, Junjie, Ruiqiang Li, Jeroen Raes, et al. "A Human Gut Microbial Gene Catalogue Established by Metagenomic Sequencing." *Nature* 464, no. 7285 (2010): 59–65. doi: 10.1038/ nature08821.

Schoenfeld, Brad J., Andrew Vigotsky, Bret Contreras, Sheona Golden, Andrew Alto, Rachel Larson, Nick Winkelman, et al. "Differential Effects of Attentional Focus Strategies During Long-Term Resistance Training." *European Journal of Sport Science* 18, no. 5 (2018): 705–712. doi: 10.1080/17461391.2018.1447020.

Seguin, Rebecca, and Miriam E. Nelson. "The Benefits of Strength Training for Older Adults." *American Journal of Preventive Medicine* 3, suppl. 2 (2003): 141–9. doi: 10.1016 /s0749-3797(03)00177-6.

Seppälä, Emma. "Connect to Thrive: Social Connection Improves Health, Well-being, and Longevity." *Psychology Today.* Accessed November 13, 2019. https://www.psychologytoday.com/us/blog/ feeling-it/201208/connect-thrive.

Sinek, Simon. *Start with Why: How Great Leaders Inspire Everyone to Take Action.* New York: Penguin Group, 2009.

Slavich, George M., Baldwin M. Way, Naomi I. Eisenberger, and Shelley E. Taylor. "Neural Sensitivity to Social Rejection is Associated with Inflammatory Responses to Social Stress." *Proceedings of the National Academy of Sciences of the United States of America* 107, no. 13 (2010): 14817-22. doi: 10.1073 /pnas.1009164107.

Snopek, Lukáš, Jiri Mlcek, Lenka Sochorova, Mojmir Baron, Irena Hlavacova, Tunde Jurikova, Rene Kizek, et al. "Contribution of Red Wine Consumption to Human Health Protection." *Molecules* 23, no. 7 (2018): 1684. doi: 10.3390/molecules23071684.

Tan, Litjen, Nancy H. Nielsen, Donald C. Young, and Zoltan Trizna for the Council on Scientific Affairs, American Medical Association. "Use of Antimicrobial Agents in Consumer Products." *Arch Dermatol* 138, no. 8 (2002): 1082–1086. doi:10.1001/archderm.138.8.1082.

U.S. Food and Drug Administration. "FDA issues final rule on safety and effectiveness of antibacterial soaps," News release, September 2, 2016. https://www.fda.gov/news-events/press-announcements/fda-issues-final-rule-safety-and-effectiveness-antibacterial-soaps.

van den Brink, Annelien C., Elske M. Brouwer-Brolsma, Agnes A. M. Berendsen, and Ondine van de Rest. "The Mediterranean, Dietary Approaches to Stop Hypertension (DASH), and Mediterranean-DASH Intervention for Neurodegenerative Delay (MIND) Diets Are Associated with Less Cognitive Decline and a Lower Risk of Alzheimer's Disease-A Review." *Advances in Nutrition* (2019): 1040–1065. doi: 10.1093/advances/nmz054.

Wang, Cai-Feng, and Ying Tian. "Reproductive Endocrine-Disrupting Effects of Triclosan: Population Exposure, Present Evidence and Potential Mechanism." *Environmental Pollution* 206 (2015): 15–201. doi: 10.1016/j.envpol.2015.07.001.

Watson, Nathaniel F., M. Safwan Badr, Gregory Belenky, Donald L. Bliwise, Orfeu M. Buxton, Daniel Buysse, David F. Dinges, et al. "Recommended Amount of Sleep for a Healthy Adult: A Joint Consensus Statement of the American Academy of Sleep Medicine and Sleep Research Society." *Sleep* 38, no. 6 (2015): 843–4. doi: 10.5665/sleep.4716.

Wu, Chenkai, Michelle. C. Odden, Gwenith G. Fisher, and Roberth S. Stawski. "Association of Retirement Age with Mortality: A Population-Based Longitudinal Study Among Older Adults in the USA." *Journal of Epidemiology and Community Health* 70, no. 9 (2016): 917–23. doi: 10.1136/jech-2015-207097.

Yang, Claire Yang, Courtney Boen, Karen Gerken, Ting Li, Kristen Schorpp, and Kathleen Mullan Harris. "Social Relationships and Physiological Determinants of Longevity Across the Human Life Span." *Proceedings of the National Academy of Sciences of the United States of America* 133, no. 3 (2016): 578–583. doi: 10.1073/pnas.1511085112.

Yeager, Ray, Daniel W. Riggs, Natasha DeJarnett, David J. Tollerud, Jeffrey Wilson, Daniel J. Conklin, Timothy E. O'Toole, et al. "Association Between Residential Greenness and Cardiovascular Disease Risk." *Journal of the American Heart Association 7*, no. 24 (2018): e009117. doi: 10.1161/JAHA.118.009117.

Zhu, Ya-qiong, Nan Peng, Ming Zhou, Pei-pei Liu, Xiao-lei Qi, Ning Wang, Gang Wang, et al. "Tai Chi and Whole-Body Vibrating Therapy in Sarcopenic Men in Advanced Old Age: A Clinical Randomized Controlled Trial." *European Journal of Ageing* 16, no. 3 (2019): 273–282. doi: 10.1007/s10433-019-00498-x.

INDEX

DNA, 6
Dynapenia, 18

E

Eggs, 41, 44
Electromagnetic frequencies
(EMFS), 111
Endorphins, 29
Environmental toxins, 111–116
Epigenetics, 6
Estrogens, 41, 44, 113–114
Exercise. *See* Movement

F

Family, 67–71
Fats, healthy, 48–49
Fernandez-Rojas, Xinia, 5
"Fight-or-flight" state, 85–86
Fish, 41, 49
Fish oil, 56
Focus meditation, 91
Forest bathing (shinrin-yoku), 96

G

Goals, 107–110
Gottman, John, 69
Gratitude, 79
Green tea, 59
Guided meditation, 91–92

H

Hand sanitizers, 112–113
Happiness, 93–94, 99
"Happy Plate," 61
Harris, Dan, 90

High intensity interval resistance training (HIIRT), 22
Hiking, 22
Hip fractures, 19
Home training, 70

I

Ikigai, 74
Incidental exercise, 26, 33
Inflammation, 39, 70, 87
Intention-setting, 78, 104–106

J

Jetton, Marge, 7, 9
Joints, 18–19, 32
Journaling, 104–105, 107–110

K

Kindness, 78–79
Kuna people, 9, 58–59

L

Lifestyle habits, 4, 87–90
Loma Linda, California, 5, 9
Love, 69, 78, 88

M

Magnesium, 56–57
Mason, Deedra, 24
Matthews, Gail, 105
Meditation, 90–92, 99
Mediterranean diet, 38–39, 41–46, 62
Melatonin, 59
Microbiome, 52–55, 62
Milk, 44
MIND diet, 47–49

ACKNOWLEDGMENTS

I acknowledge, thank, and am grateful for:

First, The Almighty, for directing me toward this opportunity and for my life's purpose.

The many people at Callisto Media who assisted in making this book possible. Special thanks to Rochelle Torke, the main editor and project leader for this book.

All my naturopathic colleagues and professors. I am proud to be part of this profession. These particular doctors inspire me daily: Dr. Millenia Lytle, a.k.a. Dr. Millie, Dr. Sean E. Heerey, Dr. Christopher SaltPaw, Dr. Saul Marcus, Dr. Sam Schikowitz, and Dr. Hatha Gbedawo.

My team whom I love. I simply could not run my practice or write this book without their support: Deblynn Gonzalez, Glenda Patterson, Erika Timar, Judy DiMaggio, Robert Notter, Larry Rogowsky, Mindy Zuckerman, and Angela Agazzi.

My Tito and Titas, both immediate and extended family members; you have assisted in setting the foundation for me.

My brother and sister-in-law: Nicholas Pimentel and Lizzy Evelyn Pimentel, owners of two world-renowned Washington, DC-based restaurants: Badsaintdc.com and Eatatelle.com.

My five beautiful and intelligent daughters who are my reason and never my excuse: Israel Zion Selassie, Maryam Makeda Selassie, Rebeca Aida Selassie, Mercy Haile Selassie, Faith Haile Selassie.

My husband, coach, spiritual adviser, and best friend, Firm Solomon Zion Selassie.

My mom for all her support and words of wisdom, Myrna Mata Pimentel.

My father, whom I hope is proud of how I have carried his legacy of healing, Dr. Ramon S. Pimentel, Jr.

ABOUT THE AUTHOR

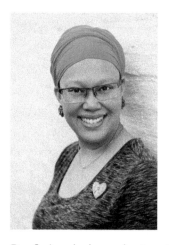

Dr. Patricia Pimentel Selassie received her naturopathic doctorate degree from Bastyr University, in Seattle, Washington. She is the founder and owner of the New Flower Center for Naturopathic Medicine in Brooklyn, New York. In her practice, Dr. Selassie blends evidence-based naturopathic medicine with listening and an intuitive coaching style so people can be their healthiest best and live their life's purpose.

Dr. Selassie is an instructor at the Open Center in NYC, has hosted over 450 live call-in nationally syndicated radio shows, is a member of the Medical Review Board for the School of Applied Functional Medicine, and is a cofounder of Nat Med Coach.

She lives with her husband and five daughters in Brooklyn, New York. She loves journaling and reading books on personal growth and development, self-help, business, and health.

Dr. Selassie is known as a doctor you can talk to. Learn more at Doctorselassie.com.

CPSIA information can be obtained
at www.ICGtesting.com
Printed in the USA
JSHW010431060320
4600JS00002B/4